300

Full-Body Body Weight Workouts Book Planner

300

Full-Body Body Weight Workouts Book Planner

Ultimate Guide to 300 Bodyweight Exercises with Step-by-Step Guides, Images, and Muscle Targeting Information for Muscle Building & Fat Loss

Be.Bull Publishing Group

Authors:

Be.Bull Publishing Group

Mauricio Vasquez

First Printing: March 2024

ISBN - 978-1-998729-18-0 (Paperback)

ISBN - 978-1-998729-19-7 (Hardcover book)

<u>TIPS</u>

- Adjust the number of repetitions and the time cap for the workouts according to your capabilities, skills and physical condition
- Listen to your body and don't push yourself too hard
- If you don't have enough space where to run, you can do jumping jacks. 100-meter run is approximately equivalent to 50 jumping jacks
- Walk into the gym with a workout already selected for you
- Get motivated with a fun workout playlist
- Put your phone on airplane mode
- Start your workout with some stretches
- Log the details of each workout so you can track your progress. You can track time and number of repetitions
- Enjoy your workouts

Dear valued customer,

Your opinion matters!

By leaving a review using the QR code provided, you can help fellow readers discover and enjoy this book. Your feedback will guide others in making informed decisions and enhance their reading experience.

Thank you for contributing to our reading community!

Mauricio

Disclaimer

FREE DOWNLOAD

BONUS - Logging Sheets of Your Workout Book

To access your free e-copy of this workout book, scan this QR code:

If you want to add more variety to your workouts, scan this QR code to check these workout books!

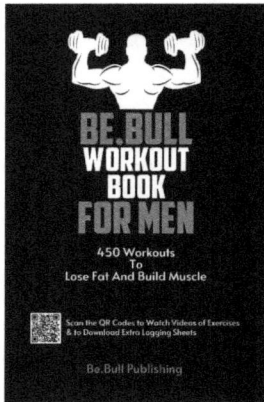

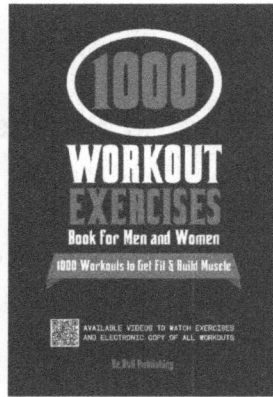

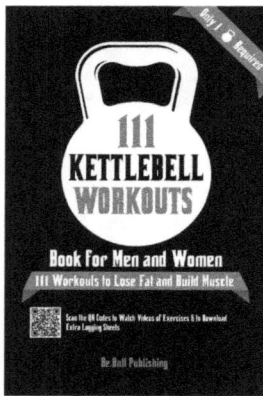

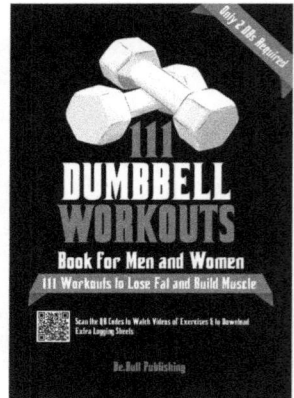

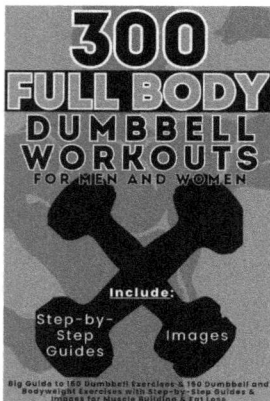

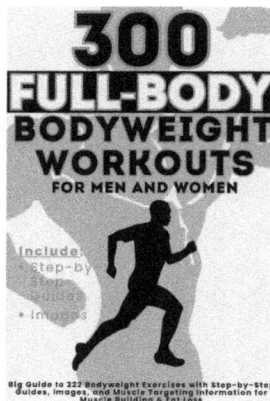

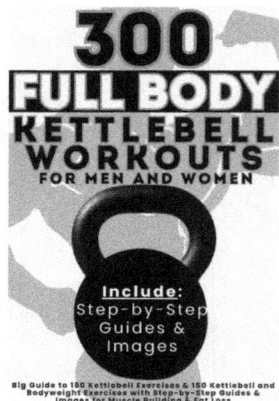

Workout	Main Muscle Groups	Instructions	Day 1	Day 2	Day 3
Workout No 1 (CrossFit) – 12-Minute AMRAP (As Many Rounds As Possible)		Complete as many rounds as possible in 12 minutes. Move fast while maintaining good form.			
10 Burpees	Full Body, Core, Cardio	Jump, drop into a push-up, jump back up. Move fast and land softly.			
15 Squats	Legs, Glutes, Core	Lower hips below knees, push through heels to rise, keep chest up.			
20 Mountain Climbers	Core, Cardio, Shoulders	In plank, drive knees toward chest, move quickly but controlled.			
Workout No 2 (HIIT) – 30 30 Intervals (4 Rounds)		30 seconds of work, 30 seconds rest per exercise. 4 total rounds.			
Jumping Jacks	Cardio, Shoulders, Core	Jump feet apart while clapping hands overhead, return to start. Move fast.			
High Knees	Cardio, Core, Legs	Run in place, drive knees high, pump arms aggressively.			
Side-to-Side Push-Ups	Chest, Triceps, Core	Do a push-up, shift to one side, push up again. Switch sides.			
Bicycle Crunches	Core, Abs, Obliques	Lie back, twist torso, bring elbow to opposite knee, extend leg.			
Workout No 3 (CrossFit) – 4 Rounds for Time		Complete 4 rounds as fast as possible. Minimal rest.			
12 Box Jumps	Legs, Glutes, Cardio	Jump onto a box, land softly, step down. Keep core tight.			
10 Pike Push-Ups	Shoulders, Triceps, Core	From downward dog position, lower head to ground, push up.			
15 Walking Lunges	Legs, Glutes, Core	Step into deep lunge, push through heel to stand, alternate legs.			
20 Flutter Kicks	Core, Lower Abs, Hip Flexors	Lie flat, keep legs straight, alternate kicking up and down.			
Workout No 4 (HIIT) – 20-Minute Tabata (20s Work, 10s Rest, 8 Rounds Per Exercise)		Alternate between 2 exercises, 20 seconds work, 10 seconds rest. 8 rounds.			
Side Plank (Left)	Core, Obliques, Shoulders	Hold plank on one side, engage core, breathe steadily. Stay straight.			
Side Plank (Right)	Core, Obliques, Shoulders	Switch sides, keep hips lifted, core tight. Breathe evenly.			
Skater Squats	Legs, Glutes, Core	Balance on one leg, squat, touch opposite hand to foot, switch sides.			
Jumping Jacks	Cardio, Shoulders, Core	Jump feet apart, clap hands overhead, return to start. Maintain rhythm.			
Workout No 5 (CrossFit) – 15-Minute Ladder (Increasing Reps Each Round)		Start with 2 reps per exercise, increase by 2 each round until 15 minutes are up.			
Squats	Legs, Glutes, Core	Lower hips below knees, drive through heels, keep chest up.			
Triceps Push-Ups	Triceps, Chest, Core	Hands under shoulders, elbows tight, lower chest to ground, push up.			
Mountain Climbers	Core, Cardio, Shoulders	Drive knees toward chest, keep core tight, move fast.			

	Workout	Main Muscle Groups	Instructions	Day 1	Day 2	Day 3
Workout No 6 (HIIT) – 10-Minute Burnout (No Rest, Max Effort)			Move continuously for 10 minutes, switch exercises every 45 seconds.			
Burpees		Full Body, Cardio, Core	Jump explosively, drop into push-up, jump back up, repeat.			
Push-Backs		Shoulders, Arms, Core	From push-up position, push hips back toward heels, return to plank.			
Russian Twists		Core, Obliques, Abs	Sit with feet lifted, twist torso side to side, touch ground beside hips.			
Workout No 7 (CrossFit) – 21-15-9 Rep Scheme			Complete 21 reps of each, then 15, then 9, as fast as possible.			
Burpees		Full Body, Cardio, Core	Drop into push-up, jump explosively, land softly, repeat.			
Reverse Crunch		Core, Lower Abs, Hip Flexors	Lift hips off floor, knees toward chest, control descent.			
Crab Toe Touch		Core, Shoulders, Coordination	In crab position, touch opposite hand to foot, switch sides.			
Workout No 8 (HIIT) – Pyramid (10-8-6-4-2 Reps)			Start with 10 reps of each, decrease by 2 each round until 2 reps.			
Inchworm		Core, Shoulders, Hamstrings	Walk hands forward to plank, hold, walk back to standing.			
Push-Up w/ Extension		Chest, Triceps, Core	Do push-up, extend one arm forward, alternate sides.			
Tuck Jumps		Legs, Core, Cardio	Jump explosively, tuck knees to chest mid-air, land softly.			
Workout No 9 (CrossFit) – 12-Minute AMRAP			Complete as many rounds as possible in 12 minutes.			
10 Step-Ups		Legs, Glutes, Core	Step onto raised surface, alternate legs, keep controlled movement.			
12 Spiderman Push-Ups		Chest, Core, Shoulders	Lower into push-up while bringing knee to elbow, alternate sides.			
15 Donkey Kicks		Glutes, Core, Balance	On hands and knees, kick leg back and up, squeeze glutes.			
Workout No 10 (HIIT) – 5-Minute Burnout Finisher			Perform 5 exercises continuously for 1 minute each. No rest.			
High Knees		Cardio, Core, Legs	Drive knees high, move fast, pump arms aggressively.			
Squats		Legs, Glutes, Core	Lower hips below knees, keep chest up, push through heels.			
Plank		Core, Shoulders, Endurance	Hold plank position, engage core, maintain straight line.			
Mountain Climbers		Core, Cardio, Shoulders	Run in place from plank, drive knees toward chest.			

	Workout	Main Muscle Groups	Instructions	Day 1	Day 2	Day 3
Workout No 11 - AMRAP 15 min			Complete as many rounds as possible in 15 minutes.			
Pull-Ups - 10 reps		Back, Arms, Core	Grip the bar, pull your chin above, and lower with control.			
Sumo Squats - 15 reps		Legs, Glutes, Core	Stand wide, toes out, squat low, keep chest up.			
High Knees - 20 reps		Legs, Cardio, Core	Run in place, lifting knees above waist level.			
Workout No 12 - HIIT - 45 sec work / 15 sec rest, 4 rounds			Perform each exercise for 45 sec, rest 15 sec, repeat 4 rounds.			
Jumping Jacks - 45 sec		Legs, Shoulders, Cardio	Jump feet apart, clap hands overhead, return.			
Push-Up w/ Extension - 45 sec		Chest, Arms, Core	Do a push-up, extend one arm forward, alternate.			
Walking Lunges - 45 sec		Legs, Glutes, Core	Step forward, drop knee to ground, switch legs.			
Plank - 45 sec		Core, Shoulders, Stability	Hold body straight on elbows, keep core engaged.			
Workout No 13 - For Time, 4 Rounds			Complete all reps as fast as possible.			
Box Jumps - 10 reps		Legs, Glutes, Cardio	Jump onto a box, land softly, step down.			
Side Plank - 12 reps per side		Core, Obliques, Stability	Hold on one side, switch after reps.			
Push-Ups - 15 reps		Chest, Arms, Core	Lower chest to floor, push back up.			
Workout No 14 - Tabata (20 sec work / 10 sec rest, 8 rounds)			Alternate exercises every round, maintain intensity.			
Bicycle Crunches - 20 sec		Core, Obliques, Abs	Alternate elbow to opposite knee.			
Side-to-Side Push-Ups - 20 sec		Chest, Core, Shoulders	Move side to side while doing push-ups.			
Workout No 15 - EMOM 12 min			Perform each exercise within the minute.			
Spiderman Push-Ups - 12 reps		Chest, Core, Arms	Bring knee to elbow as you lower down.			
Jumping Jacks - 15 reps		Legs, Shoulders, Cardio	Jump feet apart, hands overhead.			
Workout No 16 - HIIT - 50 sec work / 10 sec rest, 3 rounds			Work for 50 sec, rest 10 sec, repeat for 3 rounds.			
Tuck Jumps - 50 sec		Legs, Core, Cardio	Jump high, tuck knees to chest.			
Bear Crawl - 50 sec		Core, Shoulders, Legs	Move on all fours, keep hips low.			
Reverse Plank - 50 sec		Core, Arms, Glutes	Hold body up, face toward ceiling.			

Workout	Main Muscle Groups	Instructions	Day 1	Day 2	Day 3
Workout No 17 - 5 Rounds for Time		Complete 5 rounds quickly while maintaining form.			
Lying Leg Lifts - 15 reps	Core, Lower Abs	Lift legs straight up, lower without touching floor.			
Side Lunges - 10 reps per side	Legs, Glutes, Core	Step to side, squat low, switch sides.			
Tricep Dips - 10 reps	Arms, Triceps, Shoulders	Lower body between bars, keep elbows tight.			
Workout No 18 - HIIT - 30 sec work / 15 sec rest, 4 rounds		Perform each move for 30 sec, rest for 15 sec.			
Step-Ups - 30 sec	Legs, Glutes, Cardio	Step onto platform, alternate legs.			
Side Plank Rotation - 30 sec	Core, Shoulders, Stability	Rotate side plank, extend arm upwards.			
Squats - 30 sec	Legs, Glutes, Core	Lower hips, keep chest up, stand tall.			
Workout No 19 - 3 Rounds for Time		Complete all reps in each round quickly.			
Donkey Kicks - 12 reps per leg	Glutes, Core, Stability	Kick one leg up while keeping balance.			
Wide/Narrow Push-Ups - 10 reps	Chest, Arms, Core	Alternate between wide and narrow hand positions.			
Air Squats - 15 reps	Legs, Glutes, Core	Lower hips, explode up.			
Workout No 20 - 5 min AMRAP		Complete as many rounds as possible in 5 minutes.			
Burpees - 8 reps	Full Body, Cardio, Arms	Jump, squat, push-up, return up.			
Windshield Wipers - 12 reps	Core, Obliques, Abs	Swing legs side to side while lying.			
High Knees - 16 reps	Legs, Cardio, Core	Run in place with high knee lifts.			
Workout No 21 - AMRAP 10 min		Perform as many rounds as possible in 10 minutes.			
Burpees - 10 reps	Full Body, Cardio, Arms	Jump, squat, push-up, return up explosively.			
Side Lunges - 12 reps per leg	Legs, Glutes, Core	Step to side, squat low, switch sides.			
Russian Twists - 15 reps	Core, Obliques, Abs	Twist torso side to side while seated.			
Workout No 22 - HIIT - 40 sec work / 20 sec rest, 3 rounds		Perform each exercise for 40 sec, rest 20 sec, repeat for 3 rounds.			
Jumping Jacks - 40 sec	Legs, Shoulders, Cardio	Jump feet apart, clap hands overhead, return.			
Pike Push-Ups - 40 sec	Shoulders, Arms, Core	Hips high, lower head down, push up.			
Mountain Climbers - 40 sec	Core, Cardio, Arms	Run knees to chest from plank position.			

Workout	Main Muscle Groups	Instructions	Day 1	Day 2	Day 3
Workout No 23 - For Time, 3 Rounds		Complete all reps as fast as possible.			
Box Jumps - 12 reps	Legs, Glutes, Cardio	Jump onto a box, land softly, step down.			
Plank Rotation - 10 reps per side	Core, Shoulders, Stability	Rotate from plank, extend arm upwards.			
Push-Ups - 15 reps	Chest, Arms, Core	Lower chest to floor, push back up.			
Workout No 24 - Tabata (20 sec work / 10 sec rest, 8 rounds)		Alternate exercises every round, maintain intensity.			
Bicycle Crunches - 20 sec	Core, Obliques, Abs	Alternate elbow to opposite knee.			
Side Plank - 20 sec per side	Core, Shoulders, Stability	Hold body straight on one arm, switch sides.			
Workout No 25 - EMOM 14 min	Chest, Core, Cardio	Perform each exercise within the minute.			
Pull-Ups - 10 reps	Back, Arms, Core	Grip the bar, pull chin above, lower with control.			
Workout No 25 - Tabata (20 sec work / 10 sec rest, 8 rounds)		Alternate exercises every round, maintain intensity.			
Jump Squats - 12 reps	Legs, Glutes, Cardio	Squat down, explode up, land softly.			
Workout No 26 - HIIT - 45 sec work / 15 sec rest, 4 rounds		Work for 45 sec, rest 15 sec, repeat for 4 rounds.			
Tuck Jumps - 45 sec	Legs, Core, Cardio	Jump high, tuck knees to chest.			
Bear Crawl - 45 sec	Core, Shoulders,	Move on all fours, keep hips low.			
Reverse Plank - 45 sec	Core, Arms, Glutes	Hold body up, face toward ceiling.			
Workout No 27 - 5 Rounds for Time		Complete 5 rounds quickly while maintaining form.			
Lying Leg Lifts - 15 reps	Core, Lower Abs	Lift legs straight up, lower without touching floor.			
Side Lunges - 10 reps per side	Legs, Glutes, Core	Step to side, squat low, switch sides.			
Tricep Dips - 10 reps	Arms, Triceps, Shoulders	Lower body between bars, keep elbows tight.			
Workout No 28 - HIIT - 30 sec work / 15 sec rest, 4 rounds		Perform each move for 30 sec, rest for 15 sec.			
Step-Ups - 30 sec	Legs, Glutes, Cardio	Step onto platform, alternate legs.			
Side Plank Rotation - 30 sec	Core, Shoulders, Stability	Rotate side plank, extend arm upwards.			
Squats - 30 sec	Legs, Glutes, Core	Lower hips, keep chest up, stand tall.			
Workout No 29 - 3 Rounds for Time		Complete all reps in each round quickly.			
Donkey Kicks - 12 reps per leg	Glutes, Core, Stability	Kick one leg up while keeping balance.			
Wide/Narrow Push-Ups - 10 reps	Chest, Arms, Core	Alternate between wide and narrow hand positions.			
Air Squats - 15 reps	Legs, Glutes, Core	Lower hips, explode up.			

Workout	Main Muscle Groups	Instructions	Day 1	Day 2	Day 3
Workout No 30 - 5 min AMRAP		Complete as many rounds as possible in 5 minutes.			
Burpees - 8 reps	Full Body, Cardio, Arms	Jump, squat, push-up, return up.			
Windshield Wipers - 12 reps	Core, Obliques, Abs	Swing legs side to side while lying.			
High Knees - 16 reps	Legs, Cardio, Core	Run in place with high knee lifts.			
Workout No 31 - AMRAP 12 min		Perform as many rounds as possible in 12 minutes.			
Burpees - 10 reps	Full Body, Cardio, Arms	Jump, squat, push-up, return up explosively.			
Step-Ups - 12 reps per leg	Legs, Glutes, Core	Step onto platform, alternate legs.			
Russian Twists - 15 reps	Core, Obliques, Abs	Twist torso side to side while seated.			
Workout No 32 - HIIT - 40 sec work / 20 sec rest, 3 rounds		Perform each exercise for 40 sec, rest 20 sec, repeat for 3 rounds.			
Jumping Jacks - 40 sec	Legs, Shoulders, Cardio	Jump feet apart, clap hands overhead, return.			
Pike Push-Ups - 40 sec	Shoulders, Arms, Core	Hips high, lower head down, push up.			
Mountain Climbers - 40 sec	Core, Cardio, Arms	Run knees to chest from plank position.			
Workout No 33 - For Time, 4 Rounds		Complete all reps as fast as possible.			
Box Jumps - 12 reps	Legs, Glutes, Cardio	Jump onto a box, land softly, step down.			
Side Plank Rotation - 10 reps per side	Core, Shoulders, Stability	Rotate side plank, extend arm upwards.			
Push-Ups - 15 reps	Chest, Arms, Core	Lower chest to floor, push back up.			
Workout No 34 - Tabata (20 sec work / 10 sec rest, 8 rounds)		Alternate exercises every round, maintain intensity.			
Bicycle Crunches - 20 sec	Core, Obliques, Abs	Alternate elbow to opposite knee.			
Side Plank - 20 sec per side	Core, Shoulders, Stability	Hold body straight on one arm, switch sides.			
Workout No 35 - EMOM 14 min	Chest, Core, Cardio	Perform each exercise within the minute.			
Pull-Ups - 10 reps	Back, Arms, Core	Grip the bar, pull chin above, lower with control.			
Jump Squats - 12 reps	Legs, Glutes, Cardio	Squat down, explode up, land softly.			
Workout No 35 - HIIT - 45 sec work / 15 sec rest, 4 rounds		Work for 45 sec, rest 15 sec, repeat for 4 rounds.			
Tuck Jumps - 45 sec	Legs, Core, Cardio	Jump high, tuck knees to chest.			
Bear Crawl - 45 sec	Core, Shoulders, Legs	Move on all fours, keep hips low.			
Reverse Plank - 45 sec	Core, Arms, Glutes	Hold body up, face toward ceiling.			

Workout	Main Muscle Groups	Instructions	Day 1	Day 2	Day 3
Workout No 36 - 5 Rounds for Time		Complete 5 rounds quickly while maintaining form.			
Lying Leg Lifts - 15 reps	Core, Lower Abs	Lift legs straight up, lower without touching floor.			
Side Lunges - 10 reps per side	Legs, Glutes, Core	Step to side, squat low, switch sides.			
Tricep Dips - 10 reps	Arms, Triceps, Shoulders	Lower body between bars, keep elbows tight.			
Workout No 37 - HIIT - 30 sec work / 15 sec rest, 4 rounds		Perform each move for 30 sec, rest for 15 sec.			
Step-Ups - 30 sec	Legs, Glutes, Cardio	Step onto platform, alternate legs.			
Side Plank Rotation - 30 sec	Core, Shoulders, Stability	Rotate side plank, extend arm upwards.			
Squats - 30 sec	Legs, Glutes, Core	Lower hips, keep chest up, stand tall.			
Workout No 38 - 3 Rounds for Time		Complete all reps in each round quickly.			
Donkey Kicks - 12 reps per leg	Glutes, Core, Stability	Kick one leg up while keeping balance.			
Wide/Narrow Push-Ups - 10 reps	Chest, Arms, Core	Alternate between wide and narrow hand positions.			
Air Squats - 15 reps	Legs, Glutes, Core	Lower hips, explode up.			
Workout No 40 - 5 min AMRAP	Full Body, Core, Cardio	Complete as many rounds as possible in 5 minutes.			
Burpees - 8 reps	Full Body, Cardio, Arms	Jump, squat, push-up, return up.			
Windshield Wipers - 12 reps	Core, Obliques, Abs	Swing legs side to side while lying.			
High Knees - 16 reps	Legs, Cardio, Core	Run in place with high knee lifts.			
Workout No 39 - AMRAP 15 min		Perform as many rounds as possible in 15 minutes.			
Burpees - 12 reps	Full Body, Cardio, Arms	Jump, squat, push-up, return up explosively.			
Side Lunges - 10 reps per leg	Legs, Glutes, Core	Step to side, squat low, switch sides.			
Bicycle Crunches - 15 reps	Core, Obliques, Abs	Alternate elbow to opposite knee.			
Workout No 40 - HIIT - 45 sec work / 15 sec rest, 3 rounds		Perform each exercise for 45 sec, rest 15 sec, repeat for 3 rounds.			
Jumping Jacks - 45 sec	Legs, Shoulders, Cardio	Jump feet apart, clap hands overhead, return.			
Push-Up w/ Extension - 45 sec	Chest, Arms, Core	Do a push-up, extend one arm forward, alternate.			
Plank - 45 sec	Core, Stability, Shoulders	Hold body straight on elbows, maintain tight core.			

Workout	Main Muscle Groups	Instructions	Day 1	Day 2	Day 3
Workout No 41 - For Time, 4 Rounds		Complete all reps as fast as possible.			
Box Jumps - 12 reps	Legs, Glutes, Cardio	Jump onto a box, land softly, step down.			
Plank Rotation - 10 reps per side	Core, Shoulders, Stability	Rotate from plank, extend arm upwards.			
Push-Ups - 15 reps	Chest, Arms, Core	Lower chest to floor, push back up.			
Workout No 42 - Tabata (20 sec work / 10 sec rest, 8 rounds)		Alternate exercises every round, maintain intensity.			
Russian Twists - 20 sec	Core, Obliques, Abs	Twist torso side to side while seated.			
Side-to-Side Push-Ups - 20 sec	Chest, Core, Shoulders	Move side to side while doing push-ups.			
Workout No 45 - EMOM 12 min	Chest, Core, Cardio	Perform each exercise within the minute.			
Spiderman Push-Ups - 12 reps	Chest, Core, Arms	Bring knee to elbow as you lower down.			
Jumping Jacks - 15 reps	Legs, Shoulders, Cardio	Jump feet apart, hands overhead.			
Workout No 43 - HIIT - 50 sec work / 10 sec rest, 3 rounds		Work for 50 sec, rest 10 sec, repeat for 3 rounds.			
Tuck Jumps - 50 sec	Legs, Core, Cardio	Jump high, tuck knees to chest.			
Bear Crawl - 50 sec	Core, Shoulders, Legs	Move on all fours, keep hips low.			
Reverse Plank - 50 sec	Core, Arms, Glutes	Hold body up, face toward ceiling.			
Workout No 44 - 5 Rounds for Time		Complete 5 rounds quickly while maintaining form.			
Lying Leg Lifts - 15 reps	Core, Lower Abs	Lift legs straight up, lower without touching floor.			
Side Lunges - 10 reps per side	Legs, Glutes, Core	Step to side, squat low, switch sides.			
Tricep Dips - 10 reps	Arms, Triceps, Shoulders	Lower body between bars, keep elbows tight.			
Workout No 45 - HIIT - 30 sec work / 15 sec rest, 4 rounds		Perform each move for 30 sec, rest for 15 sec.			
Step-Ups - 30 sec	Legs, Glutes, Cardio	Step onto platform, alternate legs.			
Side Plank Rotation - 30 sec	Core, Shoulders, Stability	Rotate side plank, extend arm upwards.			
Squats - 30 sec	Legs, Glutes, Core	Lower hips, keep chest up, stand tall.			
Workout No 46 - 3 Rounds for Time		Complete all reps in each round quickly.			
Donkey Kicks - 12 reps per leg	Glutes, Core, Stability	Kick one leg up while keeping balance.			
Wide/Narrow Push-Ups - 10 reps	Chest, Arms, Core	Alternate between wide and narrow hand positions.			
Air Squats - 15 reps	Legs, Glutes, Core	Lower hips, explode up.			

Workout	Main Muscle Groups	Instructions	Day 1	Day 2	Day 3
Workout No 47 - 5 min AMRAP		Complete as many rounds as possible in 5 minutes.			
Burpees - 8 reps	Full Body, Cardio, Arms	Jump, squat, push-up, return up.			
Windshield Wipers - 12 reps	Core, Obliques, Abs	Swing legs side to side while lying.			
High Knees - 16 reps	Legs, Cardio, Core	Run in place with high knee lifts.			
Workout No 48- AMRAP 12 min		Perform as many rounds as possible in 12 minutes.			
Burpees - 12 reps	Full Body, Cardio, Arms	Jump, squat, push-up, return up explosively.			
Step-Ups - 10 reps per leg	Legs, Glutes, Core	Step onto platform, alternate legs.			
Windshield Wipers - 15 reps	Core, Obliques, Abs	Swing legs side to side while lying.			
Workout No 49- HIIT - 40 sec work / 20 sec rest, 3 rounds		Perform each exercise for 40 sec, rest 20 sec, repeat for 3 rounds.			
Jumping Jacks - 40 sec	Legs, Shoulders, Cardio	Jump feet apart, clap hands overhead, return.			
Pike Push-Ups - 40 sec	Shoulders, Arms, Core	Hips high, lower head down, push up.			
Mountain Climbers - 40 sec	Core, Cardio, Arms	Run knees to chest from plank position.			
Workout No 50- For Time, 4 Rounds		Complete all reps as fast as possible.			
Box Jumps - 12 reps	Legs, Glutes, Cardio	Jump onto a box, land softly, step down.			
Side Plank Rotation - 10 reps per side	Core, Shoulders, Stability	Rotate side plank, extend arm upwards.			
Push-Ups - 15 reps	Chest, Arms, Core	Lower chest to floor, push back up.			
Workout No 51 - Tabata (20 sec work / 10 sec rest, 8 rounds)		Alternate exercises every round, maintain intensity.			
Bicycle Crunches - 20 sec	Core, Obliques, Abs	Alternate elbow to opposite knee.			
Side Plank - 20 sec per side	Core, Shoulders, Stability	Hold body straight on one arm, switch sides.			
Workout No 55 - EMOM 14 min	Chest, Core, Cardio	Perform each exercise within the minute.			
Pull-Ups - 10 reps	Back, Arms, Core	Grip the bar, pull chin above, lower with control.			
Jump Squats - 12 reps	Legs, Glutes, Cardio	Squat down, explode up, land softly.			
Workout No 52 - HIIT - 45 sec work / 15 sec rest, 4 rounds		Work for 45 sec, rest 15 sec, repeat for 4 rounds.			
Tuck Jumps - 45 sec	Legs, Core, Cardio	Jump high, tuck knees to chest.			
Bear Crawl - 45 sec	Core, Shoulders,	Move on all fours, keep hips low.			
Reverse Plank - 45 sec	Core, Arms, Glutes	Hold body up, face toward ceiling.			

Workout	Main Muscle Groups	Instructions	Day 1	Day 2	Day 3
Workout No 53 - 5 Rounds for Time		Complete 5 rounds quickly while maintaining form.			
Lying Leg Lifts - 15 reps	Core, Lower Abs	Lift legs straight up, lower without touching floor.			
Side Lunges - 10 reps per side	Legs, Glutes, Core	Step to side, squat low, switch sides.			
Tricep Dips - 10 reps	Arms, Triceps, Shoulders	Lower body between bars, keep elbows tight.			
Workout No 54 - HIIT - 30 sec work / 15 sec rest, 4 rounds		Perform each move for 30 sec, rest for 15 sec.			
Step-Ups - 30 sec	Legs, Glutes, Cardio	Step onto platform, alternate legs.			
Side Plank Rotation - 30 sec	Core, Shoulders, Stability	Rotate side plank, extend arm upwards.			
Squats - 30 sec	Legs, Glutes, Core	Lower hips, keep chest up, stand tall.			
Workout No 55 - 3 Rounds for Time		Complete all reps in each round quickly.			
Donkey Kicks - 12 reps per leg	Glutes, Core, Stability	Kick one leg up while keeping balance.			
Wide/Narrow Push-Ups - 10 reps	Chest, Arms, Core	Alternate between wide and narrow hand positions.			
Air Squats - 15 reps	Legs, Glutes, Core	Lower hips, explode up.			
Workout No 56 - 5 min AMRAP		Complete as many rounds as possible in 5 minutes.			
Burpees - 8 reps	Full Body, Cardio, Arms	Jump, squat, push-up, return up.			
Windshield Wipers - 12 reps	Core, Obliques, Abs	Swing legs side to side while lying.			
High Knees - 16 reps	Legs, Cardio, Core	Run in place with high knee lifts.			
Workout No 57 - AMRAP 15 min		Perform as many rounds as possible in 15 minutes.			
Burpees - 12 reps	Full Body, Cardio, Arms	Jump, squat, push-up, return up explosively.			
Side Lunges - 10 reps per leg	Legs, Glutes, Core	Step to side, squat low, switch sides.			
Bicycle Crunches - 15 reps	Core, Obliques, Abs	Alternate elbow to opposite knee.			
Workout No 58 - HIIT - 45 sec work / 15 sec rest, 4 rounds		Perform each exercise for 45 sec, rest 15 sec, repeat for 4 rounds.			
Jumping Jacks - 45 sec	Legs, Shoulders, Cardio	Jump feet apart, clap hands overhead, return.			
Push-Up w/ Extension - 45 sec	Chest, Arms, Core	Do a push-up, extend one arm forward, alternate.			
Plank - 45 sec	Core, Stability, Shoulders	Hold body straight on elbows, maintain tight core.			

Workout	Main Muscle Groups	Instructions	Day 1	Day 2	Day 3
Workout No 59 - For Time, 4 Rounds		Complete all reps as fast as possible.			
Box Jumps - 12 reps	Legs, Glutes, Cardio	Jump onto a box, land softly, step down.			
Plank Rotation - 10 reps per side	Core, Shoulders, Stability	Rotate from plank, extend arm upwards.			
Push-Ups - 15 reps	Chest, Arms, Core	Lower chest to floor, push back up.			
Workout No 60 - Tabata (20 sec work / 10 sec rest, 8 rounds)		Alternate exercises every round, maintain intensity.			
Russian Twists - 20 sec	Core, Obliques, Abs	Twist torso side to side while seated.			
Side-to-Side Push-Ups - 20 sec	Chest, Core, Shoulders	Move side to side while doing push-ups.			
Workout No 61 - EMOM 12 min		Perform each exercise within the minute.			
Spiderman Push-Ups - 12 reps	Chest, Core, Arms	Bring knee to elbow as you lower down.			
Jumping Jacks - 15 reps	Legs, Shoulders, Cardio	Jump feet apart, hands overhead.			
Workout No 62 - HIIT - 50 sec work / 10 sec rest, 3 rounds		Work for 50 sec, rest 10 sec, repeat for 3 rounds.			
Tuck Jumps - 50 sec	Legs, Core, Cardio	Jump high, tuck knees to chest.			
Bear Crawl - 50 sec	Core, Shoulders, Legs	Move on all fours, keep hips low.			
Reverse Plank - 50 sec	Core, Arms, Glutes	Hold body up, face toward ceiling.			
Workout No 63 - 5 Rounds for Time		Complete 5 rounds quickly while maintaining form.			
Lying Leg Lifts - 15 reps	Core, Lower Abs	Lift legs straight up, lower without touching floor.			
Side Lunges - 10 reps per side	Legs, Glutes, Core	Step to side, squat low, switch sides.			
Tricep Dips - 10 reps	Arms, Triceps, Shoulders	Lower body between bars, keep elbows tight.			
Workout No 64 - HIIT - 30 sec work / 15 sec rest, 4 rounds		Perform each move for 30 sec, rest for 15 sec.			
Step-Ups - 30 sec	Legs, Glutes, Cardio	Step onto platform, alternate legs.			
Side Plank Rotation - 30 sec	Core, Shoulders, Stability	Rotate side plank, extend arm upwards.			
Squats - 30 sec	Legs, Glutes, Core	Lower hips, keep chest up, stand tall.			

Workout	Main Muscle Groups	Instructions	Day 1	Day 2	Day 3
Workout No 65 - 3 Rounds for Time		Complete all reps in each round quickly.			
Donkey Kicks - 12 reps per leg	Glutes, Core, Stability	Kick one leg up while keeping balance.			
Wide/Narrow Push-Ups - 10 reps	Chest, Arms, Core	Alternate between wide and narrow hand positions.			
Air Squats - 15 reps	Legs, Glutes, Core	Lower hips, explode up.			
Workout No 66 - 5 min AMRAP		Complete as many rounds as possible in 5 minutes.			
Burpees - 8 reps	Full Body, Cardio, Arms	Jump, squat, push-up, return up.			
Windshield Wipers - 12 reps	Core, Obliques, Abs	Swing legs side to side while lying.			
High Knees - 16 reps	Legs, Cardio, Core	Run in place with high knee lifts.			
Workout No 67 - AMRAP 18 min		Perform as many rounds as possible in 18 minutes.			
Box Jumps - 12 reps	Legs, Glutes, Cardio	Jump onto and off a box, land softly.			
Push-Ups - 15 reps	Chest, Arms, Core	Lower chest to floor, push back up.			
Jump Squats - 10 reps	Legs, Glutes, Core	Squat low, explode into a jump.			
Workout No 68 - HIIT - 40 sec work / 20 sec rest, 3 rounds		Perform each exercise for 40 sec, rest 20 sec, repeat.			
Bear Crawl - 40 sec	Core, Shoulders, Legs	Move forward on all fours, keep back straight.			
Plank Hold - 40 sec	Core, Stability, Shoulders	Hold body straight, tighten abs, keep position.			
Step-Ups - 40 sec	Legs, Glutes, Cardio	Step onto platform, alternate legs.			
Workout No 69 - AMRAP 14 min		Perform as many rounds as possible in 14 minutes.			
Burpees - 12 reps	Full Body, Cardio, Arms	Jump, squat, push-up, return up explosively.			
Walking Lunges - 10 reps per leg	Legs, Glutes, Core	Step forward, lower hips, alternate sides.			
Russian Twists - 20 reps	Core, Obliques, Abs	Twist torso side to side while seated.			
Workout No 70 - HIIT - 50 sec work / 10 sec rest, 3 rounds		Perform each exercise for 50 sec, rest 10 sec, repeat for 3 rounds.			
Jumping Jacks - 50 sec	Legs, Shoulders, Cardio	Jump feet apart, clap hands overhead, return.			
Pike Push-Ups - 50 sec	Shoulders, Arms, Core	Hips high, lower head down, push up.			
Mountain Climbers - 50 sec	Core, Cardio, Arms	Run knees to chest from plank position.			

Workout	Main Muscle Groups	Instructions	Day 1	Day 2	Day 3
Workout No 71 - For Time, 5 Rounds		Complete all reps as fast as possible.			
Box Jumps - 12 reps	Legs, Glutes, Cardio	Jump onto a box, land softly, step down.			
Side Plank Rotation - 10 reps per side	Core, Shoulders, Stability	Rotate side plank, extend arm upwards.			
Push-Ups - 15 reps	Chest, Arms, Core	Lower chest to floor, push back up.			
Workout No 72 - Tabata (20 sec work / 10 sec rest, 8 rounds)		Alternate exercises every round, maintain intensity.			
Bicycle Crunches - 20 sec	Core, Obliques, Abs	Alternate elbow to opposite knee.			
Side Plank - 20 sec per side	Core, Shoulders, Stability	Hold body straight on one arm, switch sides.			
Workout No 73 - EMOM 10 min		Perform each exercise within the minute.			
Pull-Ups - 8 reps	Back, Arms, Core	Grip the bar, pull chin above, lower with control.			
Jump Squats - 12 reps	Legs, Glutes, Cardio	Squat down, explode up, land softly.			
Workout No 74 - HIIT - 45 sec work / 15 sec rest, 4 rounds		Work for 45 sec, rest 15 sec, repeat for 4 rounds.			
Tuck Jumps - 45 sec	Legs, Core, Cardio	Jump high, tuck knees to chest.			
Bear Crawl - 45 sec	Core, Shoulders, Legs	Move on all fours, keep hips low.			
Reverse Plank - 45 sec	Core, Arms, Glutes	Hold body up, face toward ceiling.			
Workout No 75 - 5 Rounds for Time		Complete 5 rounds quickly while maintaining form.			
Lying Leg Lifts - 15 reps	Core, Lower Abs	Lift legs straight up, lower without touching floor.			
Side Lunges - 10 reps per side	Legs, Glutes, Core	Step to side, squat low, switch sides.			
Tricep Dips - 10 reps	Arms, Triceps, Shoulders	Lower body between bars, keep elbows tight.			
Workout No 76 - HIIT - 30 sec work / 15 sec rest, 4 rounds		Perform each move for 30 sec, rest for 15 sec.			
Step-Ups - 30 sec	Legs, Glutes, Cardio	Step onto platform, alternate legs.			
Side Plank Rotation - 30 sec	Core, Shoulders, Stability	Rotate side plank, extend arm upwards.			
Squats - 30 sec	Legs, Glutes, Core	Lower hips, keep chest up, stand tall.			

Workout	Main Muscle Groups	Instructions	Day 1	Day 2	Day 3
Workout No 77 - AMRAP 12 min		Perform as many rounds as possible in 12 minutes.			
Burpees - 10 reps	Full Body, Cardio, Arms	Jump, squat, push-up, return up explosively.			
Jump Squats - 15 reps	Legs, Glutes, Cardio	Squat down, jump high, land softly.			
Russian Twists - 20 reps	Core, Obliques, Abs	Twist torso side to side while seated.			
Workout No 78- HIIT - 45 sec work / 15 sec rest, 4 rounds		Perform each exercise for 45 sec, rest 15 sec, repeat for 4 rounds.			
Bear Crawl - 45 sec	Core, Shoulders, Legs	Move on all fours, keep hips low.			
Side Plank Rotation - 45 sec	Core, Shoulders, Stability	Rotate side plank, extend arm upwards.			
Step-Ups - 45 sec	Legs, Glutes, Cardio	Step onto platform, alternate legs.			
Workout No 79- For Time, 4 Rounds		Complete all reps as fast as possible.			
Box Jumps - 12 reps	Legs, Glutes, Cardio	Jump onto a box, land softly, step down.			
Push-Ups - 15 reps	Chest, Arms, Core	Lower chest to floor, push back up.			
Lying Leg Lifts - 15 reps	Core, Lower Abs	Lift legs straight up, lower without touching floor.			
Workout No 80 - Tabata (20 sec work / 10 sec rest, 8 rounds)		Alternate exercises every round, maintain intensity.			
Mountain Climbers - 20 sec	Core, Cardio, Arms	Run knees to chest from plank position.			
Side Lunge - 20 sec	Legs, Glutes, Core	Step to side, squat low, switch sides.			
Workout No 81 - EMOM 12 min		Perform each exercise within the minute.			
Pull-Ups - 6 reps	Back, Arms, Core	Grip the bar, pull chin above, lower with control.			
Jumping Jacks - 12 reps	Legs, Shoulders, Cardio	Jump feet apart, clap hands overhead, return.			
Workout No 82 - HIIT - 50 sec work / 10 sec rest, 3 rounds		Work for 50 sec, rest 10 sec, repeat for 3 rounds.			
Tuck Jumps - 50 sec	Legs, Core, Cardio	Jump high, tuck knees to chest.			
Side Plank - 50 sec per side	Core, Shoulders, Stability	Hold body straight on one arm, switch sides.			
Tricep Dips - 50 sec	Arms, Triceps, Shoulders	Lower body between bars, keep elbows tight.			

Workout	Main Muscle Groups	Instructions	Day 1	Day 2	Day 3
Workout No 83 - 5 Rounds for Time		Complete 5 rounds quickly while maintaining form.			
Windshield Wipers - 12 reps	Core, Obliques, Abs	Swing legs side-to-side lying down.			
Push-Ups - 15 reps	Chest, Arms, Core	Lower chest to floor, push back up.			
Squats - 15 reps	Legs, Glutes, Core	Lower hips, keep chest up, stand tall.			
Workout No 84 - HIIT - 40 sec work / 20 sec rest, 3 rounds		Perform each move for 40 sec, rest for 20 sec.			
High Knees - 40 sec	Legs, Core, Cardio	Run in place lifting knees high.			
Superman Hold - 40 sec	Core, Back, Shoulders	Extend arms and legs, hold position.			
Reverse Plank - 40 sec	Core, Arms, Glutes	Hold body up, face toward ceiling.			
Workout No 85 - AMRAP 15 min		Perform as many rounds as possible in 15 minutes.			
Lunges - 12 reps per leg	Legs, Glutes, Core	Step forward, lower hips, alternate sides.			
Pull-Ups - 8 reps	Back, Arms, Core	Grip bar, pull chin above, lower with control.			
Plank - 30 sec	Core, Stability, Shoulders	Hold body straight on elbows, maintain line.			
Workout No 86- HIIT - 30 sec work / 10 sec rest, 4 rounds		Perform each move for 30 sec, rest for 10 sec.			
Step-Ups - 30 sec	Legs, Glutes, Cardio	Step onto platform, alternate legs.			
Jump Squats - 30 sec	Legs, Glutes, Cardio	Squat down, explode up, land softly.			
Plank Rotation - 30 sec	Core, Shoulders, Stability	Rotate side plank, extend arm upwards.			
Workout No 87 HIIT (20 min AMRAP)		Complete as many rounds as possible in 20 min. Minimal rest between exercises. Maintain intensity.			
Burpees (10 reps)	Full Body, Core, Legs	Jump, squat, kick back into push-up, return up. Repeat quickly, maintaining form.			
Jumping Jacks (30 sec)	Shoulders, Legs, Core	Jump, spread feet, raise arms overhead, return to start. Maintain rhythm.			
Mountain Climbers (30 sec)	Core, Shoulders, Legs	In plank, drive knees alternately to chest at high speed. Engage core.			
Squats (15 reps)	Legs, Glutes, Core	Lower hips, keep back straight, press through heels to stand up.			
Plank Hold (30 sec)	Core, Shoulders, Arms	Maintain straight-line posture on elbows, engage core, keep hips level.			

Workout	Main Muscle Groups	Instructions	Day 1	Day 2	Day 3
Workout No 88 CrossFit (For Time, 3 Rounds)		Complete 3 rounds as quickly as possible. Rest only as needed.			
Box Jumps (12 reps)	Legs, Core, Explosiveness	Jump onto a sturdy surface, land softly, and step down to repeat.			
Push-Ups (15 reps)	Chest, Arms, Core	Lower chest to ground, push back up while keeping a straight body.			
Walking Lunges (20 reps total)	Legs, Glutes, Core	Step forward, lower hips until both knees are at 90 degrees, push back up.			
Russian Twists (30 reps total)	Core, Obliques	Sit, lean back slightly, rotate torso side to side. Keep feet off the floor for extra challenge.			
Workout No 89 HIIT (Every Minute On the Minute - EMOM, 20 Min)		Perform each exercise within the minute, rest for the remaining time.			
Burpees (12 reps)	Full Body, Core, Legs	Perform burpees as quickly as possible within 1 min. Rest for the remaining time.			
High Knees (30 sec)	Cardio, Core, Legs	Run in place, lifting knees as high as possible, maintaining speed.			
Pike Push-Ups (10 reps)	Shoulders, Arms, Core	From downward dog, lower head to floor and push back up.			
Leg Raises (15 reps)	Core, Lower Abs	Lie on back, lift legs to 90 degrees, lower slowly without touching ground.			
Workout No 90 CrossFit (5 Rounds for Time)		Complete 5 rounds as quickly as possible, minimal rest.			
Step-Ups (12 per leg)	Legs, Glutes, Core	Step onto a raised surface, drive up, alternate legs each rep.			
Wide/Narrow Push-Ups (15 reps total)	Chest, Triceps, Core	Alternate between wide and narrow grip push-ups.			
Squat Jumps (15 reps)	Legs, Explosiveness, Core	Lower into a squat, then jump explosively, landing softly.			
Side Plank (30 sec per side)	Core, Shoulders	Maintain straight line from head to feet, engage core.			
Workout No 91 HIIT (Tabata 20 sec work, 10 sec rest, 4 Rounds)		Perform each exercise for 20 seconds, rest for 10, repeat 4 rounds.			
Mountain Climbers	Core, Shoulders, Cardio	In plank, run knees towards chest rapidly.			
Squats	Legs, Glutes, Core	Lower hips, keep back straight, press through heels to stand up.			
Push-Ups	Chest, Arms, Core	Lower chest to ground, push back up while keeping a straight body.			
Jumping Jacks	Cardio, Shoulders, Legs	Jump, spread feet, raise arms overhead, return to start.			

Workout	Main Muscle Groups	Instructions	Day 1	Day 2	Day 3
Workout No 92 CrossFit (Chipper Complete 1 Round for Time)		Complete all reps in order as quickly as possible.			
Burpees (30 reps)	Full Body, Core, Legs	Jump, squat, kick back into push-up, return up.			
Lunges (20 per leg)	Legs, Glutes, Core	Step forward, lower hips, push back up.			
Plank to Push-Up (20 reps)	Core, Shoulders, Arms	Start in plank, transition to push-up position, alternate arms.			
Jump Squats (25 reps)	Legs, Core, Cardio	Lower into squat, explode up into jump, land softly.			
Workout No 93 HIIT (Time-Based, 18 min EMOM)		Perform each exercise within the minute, rest as needed.			
Burpees (10 reps)	Full Body, Core, Legs	Perform burpees as quickly as possible within 1 min.			
High Knees (30 sec)	Cardio, Core, Legs	Run in place, lifting knees as high as possible.			
Side Plank (30 sec per side)	Core, Shoulders	Maintain straight line from head to feet, engage core.			
Jump Squats (12 reps)	Legs, Core, Cardio	Lower into squat, explode up into jump, land softly.			
Workout No 94 CrossFit (For Time, 4 Rounds)		Complete 4 rounds as quickly as possible.			
Box Jumps (10 reps)	Legs, Core, Explosiveness	Jump onto a sturdy surface, land softly, and step down to repeat.			
Tricep Dips (15 reps)	Arms, Chest, Core	Lower body between bars, push back up.			
Side Lunges (12 per leg)	Legs, Glutes, Core	Step laterally, bend knee, return to standing.			
V-Ups (15 reps)	Core, Lower Abs	Lie on back, lift legs and torso simultaneously, forming a 'V'.			
Workout No 95 (CrossFit) - AMRAP 12 Min		Complete as many rounds as possible in 12 minutes.			
Burpees - 10 reps	Full Body, Cardio, Core	Jump, squat down, kick back into a push-up, return up, and repeat. Keep a steady pace.			
Jumping Jacks - 20 reps	Cardio, Legs, Core	Jump to spread legs and clap hands overhead, then return to start. Maintain a steady rhythm.			
Push-Ups - 10 reps	Chest, Shoulders, Core	Lower your body to the ground and push up. Maintain a straight line from head to heels.			
Lunges - 10 reps each leg	Legs, Core, Balance	Step forward, lower hips to drop knee to the ground, return to standing, and alternate legs.			

Workout	Main Muscle Groups	Instructions	Day 1	Day 2	Day 3
Workout No 96 (HIIT) - 30s Work / 15s Rest x 4 Rounds		Perform each exercise for 30 seconds, rest 15 seconds, complete 4 rounds.			
High Knees	Cardio, Core, Legs	Run in place lifting knees high, maintaining a fast pace.			
Mountain Climbers	Core, Shoulders, Cardio	Run in plank position, bringing knees towards chest quickly.			
Squats	Legs, Core, Glutes	Bend knees to lower body, keeping back straight and chest up.			
Plank Hold	Core, Shoulders, Stability	Hold a plank position on elbows, maintaining a tight core.			
Workout No 97 (CrossFit) - For Time		Complete the workout as fast as possible.			
Burpees - 20 reps	Full Body, Cardio, Core	Jump, squat down, kick back into a push-up, return up, and repeat.			
Step-Ups - 20 reps	Legs, Core, Glutes	Step onto a raised platform, alternate legs each step.			
Push-Ups - 15 reps	Chest, Shoulders, Core	Lower chest to the floor, then push back up.			
Sit-Ups - 20 reps	Core, Stability, Strength	Lie down, sit up fully, and lower back to start position.			
Workout No 98 (HIIT) - 40s Work / 20s Rest x 3 Rounds		Perform each exercise for 40 seconds, rest 20 seconds, complete 3 rounds.			
Squat Jumps	Legs, Cardio, Core	Perform a deep squat, jump up explosively, and land softly.			
Russian Twists	Core, Obliques, Stability	Twist torso holding weight, seated on the ground.			
Side Plank (Each Side)	Core, Stability, Shoulders	Hold a side plank on one arm, switch sides halfway through.			
Flutter Kicks	Core, Lower Abs, Hip Flexors	Lie on back, alternate kicking legs in small, rapid motion.			
Workout No 99 (CrossFit) - 15-Minute EMOM		Every minute on the minute, perform the assigned exercises.			
Tuck Jumps - 10 reps	Legs, Cardio, Explosiveness	Jump high, tuck knees to chest mid-air, land softly.			
Plank to Push-Up - 10 reps	Core, Shoulders, Arms	Transition from a plank to a push-up and return.			
Lunges - 12 reps	Legs, Core, Stability	Step forward, lower hips, alternate legs each step.			
Bear Crawl - 15 meters	Core, Shoulders, Coordination	Crawl forward on all fours, keeping hips low.			

Workout	Main Muscle Groups	Instructions	Day 1	Day 2	Day 3
Workout No 100 (HIIT) - 45s Work / 15s Rest x 3 Rounds		Perform each exercise for 45 seconds, rest 15 seconds, complete 3 rounds.			
Jumping Jacks	Cardio, Legs, Core	Jump to spread legs and clap hands overhead.			
Burpees	Full Body, Cardio, Core	Jump, squat, push-up, and return to standing.			
Side-to-Side Push-Ups	Chest, Core, Shoulders	Move sideways between each push-up to engage the core.			
Wall Sit	Legs, Core, Stability	Sit against a wall, holding thighs parallel to the floor.			
Workout No 101 (CrossFit) - AMRAP 10 Min		Complete as many rounds as possible in 10 minutes.			
Box Jumps - 15 reps	Legs, Cardio, Explosiveness	Jump onto and off a box repeatedly, landing softly.			
Push-Ups - 12 reps	Chest, Shoulders, Arms	Lower chest to the ground, then push back up.			
Plank Rotation - 10 reps	Core, Shoulders, Stability	Rotate in plank position, extending one arm upward, switch sides.			
Russian Twists - 15 reps	Core, Obliques, Stability	Twist torso while seated, keeping feet off the ground.			
Workout No 102 (HIIT) - 30s Work / 10s Rest x 5 Rounds		Perform each exercise for 30 seconds, rest 10 seconds, complete 5 rounds.			
High Knees	Cardio, Core, Legs	Run in place, lifting knees high, maintaining a fast pace.			
Squats	Legs, Core, Glutes	Bend knees to lower body, keeping back straight.			
Side Lunges	Legs, Core, Stability	Step sideways into a lunge, alternating legs.			
Plank Hold	Core, Shoulders, Stability	Hold a plank position on elbows, maintaining a tight core.			
Workout No 103 (CrossFit) - For Time		Complete the workout as fast as possible.			
Burpees - 25 reps	Full Body, Cardio, Core	Jump, squat down, kick back into a push-up, return up.			
Squats - 30 reps	Legs, Core, Glutes	Bend knees to lower body, keeping back straight.			
Push-Ups - 20 reps	Chest, Shoulders, Core	Lower body to the ground and push up.			
Sit-Ups - 25 reps	Core, Stability, Strength	Lie down, sit up fully, and lower back to start position.			
Workout No 104 (HIIT) - Tabata 20s Work / 10s Rest x 8 Rounds		Perform each exercise for 20 seconds, rest 10 seconds, complete 8 rounds.			
Burpees	Full Body, Cardio, Core	Jump, squat, push-up, and return to standing.			
Jumping Jacks	Cardio, Legs, Core	Jump to spread legs and clap hands overhead.			
Push-Ups	Chest, Shoulders, Arms	Lower chest to the ground, then push back up.			
Plank Hold	Core, Shoulders, Stability	Hold a plank position on elbows, maintaining a tight core.			

Workout	Main Muscle Groups	Instructions	Day 1	Day 2	Day 3
Workout No 105 (CrossFit) - AMRAP 12 min		Perform as many rounds as possible in 12 min. Maintain good form throughout.			
10 Burpees	Legs, Chest, Core	Jump, squat, kick back into push-up, return up. Keep pace and breathe.			
15 Push-Ups	Chest, Arms, Core	Lower chest to the ground, keep elbows tucked, push up.			
20 Squats	Legs, Glutes, Core	Keep feet shoulder-width apart, lower hips, maintain upright torso.			
Workout No 106 (HIIT) - 30s Work / 15s Rest (4 Rounds)		Perform each exercise for 30 seconds, rest 15 seconds, repeat 4 times.			
Jumping Jacks	Legs, Arms, Cardio	Jump, spread legs, clap hands overhead. Maintain pace.			
Mountain Climbers	Core, Shoulders, Legs	Run in place in plank position, drive knees to chest.			
Side-to-Side Push-Ups	Chest, Core, Arms	Shift side-to-side during push-ups, engaging core.			
High Knees	Legs, Cardio, Core	Run in place lifting knees high, keeping an upright posture.			
Workout No 107 (CrossFit) - 5 Rounds for Time		Complete 5 rounds as fast as possible, maintaining form.			
15 V-Ups	Core, Hip Flexors, Legs	Lie back, lift legs and torso, touch hands to toes.			
20 Lunge Steps	Legs, Glutes, Core	Step forward, lower hips to drop knee to ground.			
Workout No 108 (HIIT) - 20s Work / 10s Rest (Tabata Style)		Perform 8 rounds per exercise, 20s work, 10s rest.			
Tuck Jumps	Legs, Core, Cardio	Jump high, tuck knees to chest mid-air, land softly.			
Push-Ups w/ Extension	Chest, Core, Arms	Perform push-up, extend one arm forward, alternate.			
Workout No 109 Time-Based CrossFit AMRAP (15 min)		Perform as many rounds as possible in 15 min: 10 Burpees, 15 Squats, 20 Mountain Climbers. Rest as needed but keep moving.			
10 Burpees	Chest, Shoulders, Legs	Jump, squat down, kick back into push-up, return up. Perform explosively and maintain pace.			
15 Squats	Legs, Core, Glutes	Stand tall, lower hips down, keep chest up, push through heels to stand.			
20 Mountain Climbers	Core, Shoulders, Legs	Maintain plank, drive knees toward chest rapidly, keeping core engaged.			

Workout	Main Muscle Groups	Instructions	Day 1	Day 2	Day 3
Workout No 110 Rep-Based CrossFit Chipper		Complete all reps for each movement before moving on: 50 Jumping Jacks, 40 Russian Twists, 30 Push-Ups, 20 Box Jumps, 10 Burpees.			
50 Jumping Jacks	Legs, Shoulders, Core	Jump to spread legs, raise hands overhead, return to start.			
40 Russian Twists	Obliques, Core, Shoulders	Seated, rotate torso side-to-side while keeping core tight.			
30 Push-Ups	Chest, Shoulders, Core	Lower body to ground, push up, keep core engaged.			
20 Box Jumps	Legs, Glutes, Core	Jump onto and off a stable surface, land softly.			
10 Burpees	Chest, Shoulders, Legs	Jump, squat down, kick back into push-up, return up.			
Workout No 111 CrossFit EMOM (Every Minute On the Minute for 12 min)		Perform the set number of reps every minute, rest for the remainder: 10 Lunge, 10 Pike Push-Up, 10 Flutter Kicks.			
10 Lunge	Legs, Glutes, Core	Step forward, lower back knee toward floor, push back up.			
10 Pike Push-Up	Shoulders, Chest, Triceps	Hinge at hips into pike position, lower head to floor, push back up.			
10 Flutter Kicks	Core, Hip Flexors, Legs	Lie on back, alternately kick legs up and down rapidly.			
Workout No 112 CrossFit Tabata (20 sec work, 10 sec rest, 4 rounds)		Perform 4 rounds: 20 sec High Knees, 10 sec rest, 20 sec Side Plank, 10 sec rest, 20 sec Squats, 10 sec rest.			
20 sec High Knees	Legs, Core, Cardiovascular	Run in place lifting knees high, maintain a steady pace.			
20 sec Side Plank (each side)	Core, Obliques, Shoulders	Support body on one elbow, keep body aligned.			
20 sec Squats	Legs, Glutes, Core	Lower hips down, keep chest up, push through heels to stand.			
Workout No 5 CrossFit Pyramid	Full Body	Increase then decrease reps: 5, 10, 15, 10, 5 reps of Push-Ups, Lying Leg Lifts, Skater Squats.			
Push-Ups	Chest, Shoulders, Core	Lower chest to floor, push up, maintain straight posture.			
Lying Leg Lifts	Core, Hip Flexors, Lower Abs	Lift legs up together, control descent, keep lower back down.			
Skater Squats	Legs, Glutes, Core	Balance on one leg, squat, touch opposite hand to foot.			

Workout	Main Muscle Groups	Instructions	Day 1	Day 2	Day 3
Workout No 113 20-Min HIIT Circuit		Perform each exercise for 45 sec, rest 15 sec: Burpees, Side Lunge, Plank Rotations, Triceps Dips, Jumping Jacks.			
Burpees	Chest, Shoulders, Legs	Jump, squat down, kick back into push-up, return up.			
Side Lunge	Legs, Glutes, Core	Step sideways, keep one leg straight, lower into lunge.			
Plank Rotations	Core, Shoulders, Obliques	Hold plank, rotate torso, extend arm upwards, switch sides.			
Triceps Dips	Triceps, Shoulders, Core	Dip body between two bars or a chair, keeping elbows tucked.			
Jumping Jacks	Legs, Shoulders, Cardiovascular	Jump to spread legs, raise hands overhead, return to start.			
Workout No 114 HIIT AMRAP (As Many Rounds As Possible in 12 min)		Repeat as many rounds as possible in 12 min: 10 Tuck Jumps, 15 Push-Ups, 20 Mountain Climbers.			
10 Tuck Jumps	Legs, Core, Cardiovascular	Jump explosively, bring knees to chest mid-air.			
15 Push-Ups	Chest, Shoulders, Core	Lower chest to floor, push up, maintain posture.			
20 Mountain Climbers	Core, Shoulders, Legs	Drive knees towards chest in a plank position.			
Workout No 115 30-Second Interval HIIT		Perform each for 30 sec, rest 10 sec: Wall Sit, Fire Hydrant, Star Plank, Dolphin Kick.			
Wall Sit	Legs, Glutes, Core	Sit against a wall, legs at 90-degree angle, hold.			
Fire Hydrant	Glutes, Hips, Core	On hands/knees, lift leg to side, keep knee bent.			
Star Plank	Core, Shoulders, Glutes	Extend arms and legs outward in a plank position.			
Dolphin Kick	Lower Back, Glutes, Core	Lie face down, kick legs like a dolphin tail.			
Workout No 116 HIIT Ladder		Increase reps each round: 5, 10, 15, 20 reps of Reverse Crunch, Calf Raise, Superman.			
Reverse Crunch	Core, Lower Abs, Hip Flexors	Lift hips off floor, knees towards chest, control descent.			
Calf Raise	Calves, Ankles, Balance	Lift heels off the ground, balance on toes, lower slowly.			
Superman	Lower Back, Core, Glutes	Extend arms and legs while face down, hold position.			
Workout No 117 Full-Body HIIT Burn		Perform 40 sec work, 20 sec rest for 3 rounds: Crab Walk, Squats, V-Ups, Step Ups.			
Crab Walk	Core, Shoulders, Glutes	Walk backward on hands and feet, hips elevated.			
Squats	Legs, Glutes, Core	Lower hips down, keep chest up, push through heels.			
V-Ups	Core, Abs, Hip Flexors	Lift legs and torso together, forming a 'V' shape.			
Step Ups	Legs, Glutes, Core	Step onto a raised surface, alternate legs, maintain control.			

Workout	Main Muscle Groups	Instructions	Day 1	Day 2	Day 3
Workout No 123 HIIT AMRAP (As Many Rounds As Possible in 12 min)		Repeat rounds in 12 min: 10 Lying Leg Lifts, 12 Push-Ups, 15 Skater Squats.			
10 Lying Leg Lifts	Core, Hip Flexors, Lower Abs	Lift legs together, control descent, keep lower back down.			
12 Push-Ups	Chest, Shoulders, Core	Lower chest to floor, push up, keep core engaged.			
15 Skater Squats	Legs, Glutes, Core	Balance on one leg, squat, touch opposite hand to foot.			
Workout No 124 30-Second Interval HIIT		Perform each for 30 sec, rest 10 sec: Crab Walk, Side Lunge, Dolphin Kick, V-Ups.			
Crab Walk	Core, Shoulders, Glutes	Walk backward on hands and feet, hips elevated.			
Side Lunge	Legs, Glutes, Core	Step sideways, keep one leg straight, lower into lunge.			
Dolphin Kick	Lower Back, Glutes, Core	Lie face down, kick legs like a dolphin tail.			
V-Ups	Core, Abs, Hip Flexors	Lift legs and torso together, forming a 'V' shape.			
Workout No 125 HIIT Ladder		Increase reps each round: 5, 10, 15, 20 reps of Windshield Wipers, Single Leg Squat, Superman.			
Windshield Wipers	Core, Obliques, Lower Back	Swing legs side-to-side lying down, control movement.			
Single Leg Squat	Legs, Glutes, Core	Stand on one leg, squat down, maintain balance.			
Superman	Lower Back, Core, Glutes	Extend arms and legs while face down, hold position.			
Workout No 126 Full-Body HIIT Burn		Perform 40 sec work, 20 sec rest for 3 rounds: Inchworm, Squats, Bird Dog, Jumping Jacks.			
Inchworm	Shoulders, Core, Hamstrings	Walk hands forward from standing, hold plank, walk back.			
Squats	Legs, Glutes, Core	Lower hips down, keep chest up, push through heels.			
Bird Dog	Core, Lower Back, Balance	Extend opposite arm and leg from kneeling position.			
Jumping Jacks	Legs, Shoulders, Cardiovascular	Jump to spread legs, raise hands overhead, return to start.			
Workout No 127 (CrossFit) – 15-Minute AMRAP		Complete as many rounds as possible in 15 minutes. Move fast but maintain good form.			
10 Burpees	Full Body, Core, Cardio	Start standing, drop into a squat, kick feet back, do a push-up, jump back up explosively.			
15 Squats	Legs, Core, Glutes	Stand shoulder-width apart, lower hips below knees, keep chest up, push through heels to rise.			
10 Push-Ups	Chest, Triceps, Core	Lower chest to the ground, keep elbows at 45-degree angle, push back up. Maintain core tight.			
20 Mountain Climbers	Core, Cardio, Shoulders	In plank position, drive knees toward chest rapidly. Keep back straight, move at high intensity.			

Workout	Main Muscle Groups	Instructions	Day 1	Day 2	Day 3
Workout No 128 (HIIT) – 30 30 Intervals (5 Rounds)		30 seconds work, 30 seconds rest per exercise. Complete 5 rounds. Maintain intensity.			
Jumping Jacks	Cardio, Shoulders, Core	Jump feet apart while clapping hands overhead, then return to start. Keep pace high.			
High Knees	Cardio, Core, Legs	Run in place, drive knees up to waist height. Engage core and pump arms.			
Side-to-Side Push-Up	Chest, Triceps, Core	Perform a push-up, shift weight to one side, push up again. Alternate sides.			
Bicycle Crunches	Core, Abs, Obliques	Lie on back, twist torso to bring elbow to opposite knee, extend opposite leg.			
Workout No 129 (CrossFit) – 4 Rounds for Time		Complete 4 rounds as fast as possible. Rest only as needed.			
12 Box Jumps	Legs, Glutes, Cardio	Jump explosively onto a box or sturdy surface, land softly, stand up fully, step down.			
10 Pike Push-Ups	Shoulders, Triceps, Core	In downward dog position, lower head towards ground, push up. Keep elbows tucked.			
15 Walking Lunges	Legs, Glutes, Core	Step forward into a deep lunge, drive through heel, alternate legs, maintain upright posture.			
20 Flutter Kicks	Core, Lower Abs, Hip Flexors	Lie flat, alternate kicking legs up and down without touching ground, keep core tight.			
Workout No 130 (HIIT) – EMOM (Every Minute on the Minute) for 12 Minutes		Start a new movement at the beginning of each minute. Complete reps, then rest until next minute.			
8 Burpees	Full Body, Cardio, Core	Drop into a push-up, jump feet back, explode up into a jump, land softly.			
10 Push-Backs	Shoulders, Arms, Core	From push-up position, push hips back toward heels, then return to plank.			
15 Russian Twists	Core, Obliques, Abs	Sit with feet lifted, twist torso side to side, touch ground beside hips.			
Workout No 131 (HIIT) – 20-Minute Tabata (20s Work, 10s Rest)		8 Rounds of 4 Exercises (20s on, 10s rest). Keep intensity high.			
Side Plank (Left)	Core, Obliques, Shoulders	Hold body in straight line, engage core, support weight on one forearm.			
Side Plank (Right)	Core, Obliques, Shoulders	Hold on opposite side, maintain stability, breathe evenly.			
Skater Squats	Legs, Glutes, Core	Balance on one leg, squat down, touch opposite hand to foot, alternate sides.			
Jumping Jacks	Cardio, Shoulders, Core	Jump feet apart while clapping hands overhead, then return to start.			

Workout	Main Muscle Groups	Instructions	Day 1	Day 2	Day 3
Workout No 132 (CrossFit) – 21-15-9 Reps Scheme		Perform 21 reps of each, then 15, then 9, as fast as possible.			
Burpees	Full Body, Cardio, Core	Drop into push-up, jump explosively, repeat.			
Reverse Crunch	Core, Lower Abs, Hip Flexors	Lift hips off floor, knees toward chest, control descent.			
Crab Toe Touch	Core, Shoulders, Coordination	In crab position, touch opposite hand to foot, alternate sides.			
Workout No 133 (HIIT) – Pyramid (10-8-6-4-2 Reps)		Start with 10 reps of each, decrease by 2 each round until you reach 2 reps.			
Inchworm	Core, Shoulders, Hamstrings	Walk hands forward to plank, hold, walk back to standing.			
Push-Up w/ Extension	Chest, Triceps, Core	Do a push-up, extend one arm forward, alternate sides.			
Tuck Jumps	Legs, Core, Cardio	Jump explosively, tuck knees to chest mid-air, land softly.			
Workout No 134 (CrossFit) – 12-Minute AMRAP		Complete as many rounds as possible in 12 minutes.			
10 Step-Ups	Legs, Glutes, Core	Step onto raised surface, alternate legs, keep controlled movement.			
12 Spiderman Push-Ups	Chest, Core, Shoulders	Lower into push-up while bringing knee to elbow, alternate sides.			
15 Donkey Kicks	Glutes, Core, Balance	On hands and knees, kick leg back and up, squeeze glutes.			
Workout No 135 (HIIT) – 5-Minute Burnout Finisher		Perform 5 exercises continuously for 1 minute each. No rest.			
High Knees	Cardio, Core, Legs	Drive knees high, move fast, pump arms.			
Squats	Legs, Glutes, Core	Lower hips below knees, keep chest up, push through heels.			
Plank	Core, Shoulders, Endurance	Hold plank position, engage core, maintain straight line.			
Mountain Climbers	Core, Cardio, Shoulders	Run in place from plank, drive knees toward chest.			
Jumping Jacks	Cardio, Shoulders, Core	Jump feet apart, clap hands overhead, return to start.			
Workout No 136 (CrossFit) – 12-Minute AMRAP (As Many Rounds As Possible)		Complete as many rounds as possible in 12 minutes. Maintain good form while keeping intensity high.			
10 Burpees	Full Body, Core, Cardio	Jump up, drop into a squat, kick feet back into a push-up, return up and repeat explosively.			
12 Squats	Legs, Glutes, Core	Lower hips below knees, chest up, drive through heels to stand. Keep steady pace.			
15 Mountain Climbers (Each Side)	Core, Cardio, Shoulders	In plank, drive knees toward chest rapidly, keeping core tight and moving continuously.			
10 Push-Ups	Chest, Triceps, Core	Lower body to ground, keep elbows at 45 degrees, push up while keeping core engaged.			

Workout	Main Muscle Groups	Instructions	Day 1	Day 2	Day 3
Workout No 137 (HIIT) – 30 30 Intervals (5 Rounds)		30 seconds of work, 30 seconds of rest per exercise. Complete 5 rounds.			
Jumping Jacks	Cardio, Shoulders, Core	Jump feet apart while clapping hands overhead, then return to start. Keep high intensity.			
High Knees	Cardio, Core, Legs	Drive knees high, run in place fast, engage core and pump arms.			
Side-to-Side Push-Ups	Chest, Triceps, Core	Perform a push-up, shift to one side, push up again, alternate sides.			
Bicycle Crunches	Core, Abs, Obliques	Lie on back, twist torso to bring elbow to opposite knee, extend opposite leg.			
Workout No 138 (CrossFit) – 5 Rounds for Time		Complete 5 rounds as fast as possible, keeping form strict. Rest only if needed.			
10 Box Jumps	Legs, Glutes, Cardio	Jump explosively onto a box, land softly, step down, and repeat quickly.			
10 Pike Push-Ups	Shoulders, Triceps, Core	In downward dog position, lower head toward ground, push up. Keep core engaged.			
12 Walking Lunges	Legs, Glutes, Core	Step forward into deep lunge, push through heel to stand, alternate legs.			
15 Flutter Kicks	Core, Lower Abs, Hip Flexors	Lie on back, keep legs straight, alternate kicking up and down. Keep lower back pressed down.			
Workout No 139 (HIIT) – 20-Minute Tabata (20s Work, 10s Rest, 8 Rounds Per Exercise)		Alternate between 2 exercises, doing 20 seconds of work followed by 10 seconds of rest. Repeat each pair for 8 rounds.			
Side Plank (Left)	Core, Obliques, Shoulders	Hold plank on one side, engage core, breathe steadily. Maintain a straight body line.			
Side Plank (Right)	Core, Obliques, Shoulders	Switch to opposite side and hold. Keep hips lifted, maintain steady breathing.			
Skater Squats	Legs, Glutes, Core	Balance on one leg, squat down, touch opposite hand to foot, then switch sides.			
Jumping Jacks	Cardio, Shoulders, Core	Jump feet apart, clap hands overhead, return to start. Keep pace fast.			
Workout No 140 (CrossFit) – 15-Minute Ladder (Increasing Reps Each Round)		Start with 2 reps of each movement, increase by 2 reps per round until 15 minutes are up.			
Squats	Legs, Glutes, Core	Lower hips below knees, drive through heels, keep chest up.			
Triceps Push-Ups	Triceps, Chest, Core	Hands under shoulders, elbows tight, lower chest to ground, push up.			
Mountain Climbers	Core, Cardio, Shoulders	In plank, drive knees towards chest quickly, keeping pace high.			

Workout	Main Muscle Groups	Instructions	Day 1	Day 2	Day 3
Workout No 141 (HIIT) – 10-Minute Burnout (No Rest, Max Effort)		Move continuously for 10 minutes, switching exercises every 45 seconds.			
Burpees	Full Body, Cardio, Core	Jump explosively, drop into push-up, jump back up, repeat continuously.			
Push-Backs	Shoulders, Arms, Core	From push-up position, push hips back toward heels, return to plank.			
Russian Twists	Core, Obliques, Abs	Sit with feet lifted, twist torso side to side, touch ground beside hips.			
Workout No 142 (CrossFit) – 21-15-9 Rep Scheme		Complete 21 reps of each, then 15, then 9, as fast as possible.			
Burpees	Full Body, Cardio, Core	Drop into a push-up, jump explosively, land softly, and repeat.			
Reverse Crunch	Core, Lower Abs, Hip Flexors	Lift hips off floor, knees towards chest, control descent.			
Crab Toe Touch	Core, Shoulders, Coordination	In crab position, touch opposite hand to foot, alternate sides.			
Workout No 143 (HIIT) – Pyramid (10-8-6-4-2 Reps)		Start with 10 reps of each, decrease by 2 each round until you reach 2 reps.			
Inchworm	Core, Shoulders, Hamstrings	Walk hands forward to plank, hold, walk back to standing.			
Push-Up w/ Extension	Chest, Triceps, Core	Perform push-up, extend one arm forward, alternate sides.			
Tuck Jumps	Legs, Core, Cardio	Jump explosively, tuck knees to chest mid-air, land softly.			
Workout No 144 (CrossFit) – 12-Minute AMRAP		Complete as many rounds as possible in 12 minutes.			
10 Step-Ups	Legs, Glutes, Core	Step onto raised surface, alternate legs, keep controlled movement.			
12 Spiderman Push-Ups	Chest, Core, Shoulders	Lower into push-up while bringing knee to elbow, alternate sides.			
15 Donkey Kicks	Glutes, Core, Balance	On hands and knees, kick leg back and up, squeeze glutes.			
Workout No 145 (HIIT) – 5-Minute Burnout Finisher		Perform 5 exercises continuously for 1 minute each. No rest.			
High Knees	Cardio, Core, Legs	Drive knees high, move fast, pump arms.			
Squats	Legs, Glutes, Core	Lower hips below knees, keep chest up, push through heels.			
Plank	Core, Shoulders, Endurance	Hold plank position, engage core, maintain straight line.			
Mountain Climbers	Core, Cardio, Shoulders	Run in place from plank, drive knees toward chest.			
Jumping Jacks	Cardio, Shoulders, Core	Jump feet apart, clap hands overhead, return to start.			

Workout	Main Muscle Groups	Instructions	Day 1	Day 2	Day 3
Workout No 146 (CrossFit) – 15-Minute AMRAP		Complete as many rounds as possible in 15 minutes. Maintain intensity while keeping good form.			
10 Burpees	Full Body, Core, Cardio	Jump, drop into a push-up, jump back up explosively. Maintain steady rhythm and control.			
15 Squats	Legs, Glutes, Core	Stand shoulder-width apart, lower hips below knees, push through heels to rise. Keep chest up.			
10 Push-Ups	Chest, Triceps, Core	Lower chest to ground, keep elbows at 45 degrees, push up while keeping core tight.			
20 Mountain Climbers	Core, Cardio, Shoulders	In plank position, drive knees toward chest quickly. Engage core throughout.			
Workout No 147 (HIIT) – 30 30 Intervals (4 Rounds)		30 seconds of work, 30 seconds of rest per exercise. Complete 4 rounds.			
Jumping Jacks	Cardio, Shoulders, Core	Jump feet apart while clapping hands overhead, return to start. Keep pace high.			
High Knees	Cardio, Core, Legs	Run in place, drive knees up to waist height. Engage core and pump arms.			
Side-to-Side Push-Ups	Chest, Triceps, Core	Perform push-up, shift to one side, push up again. Alternate sides.			
Bicycle Crunches	Core, Abs, Obliques	Lie on back, twist torso to bring elbow to opposite knee, extend opposite leg.			
Workout No 148 (CrossFit) – 4 Rounds for Time		Complete 4 rounds as fast as possible. Rest only as needed.			
12 Box Jumps	Legs, Glutes, Cardio	Jump explosively onto a box, land softly, stand up fully, step down.			
10 Pike Push-Ups	Shoulders, Triceps, Core	In downward dog position, lower head toward ground, push up. Keep core engaged.			
15 Walking Lunges	Legs, Glutes, Core	Step forward into a deep lunge, push through heel, alternate legs.			
20 Flutter Kicks	Core, Lower Abs, Hip Flexors	Lie flat, keep legs straight, alternate kicking up and down. Maintain tight core.			
Workout No 149 (HIIT) – EMOM (Every Minute on the Minute) for 12 Minutes		Start a new movement at the beginning of each minute. Complete reps, then rest until next minute.			
8 Burpees	Full Body, Cardio, Core	Drop into push-up, jump feet back, explode up into a jump, land softly.			
10 Push-Backs	Shoulders, Arms, Core	From push-up position, push hips back toward heels, then return to plank.			
15 Russian Twists	Core, Obliques, Abs	Sit with feet lifted, twist torso side to side, touch ground beside hips.			

Workout	Main Muscle Groups	Instructions	Day 1	Day 2	Day 3
Workout No 150 (CrossFit) – 10-Minute Ladder (Increasing Reps Each Round)		Start with 2 reps per exercise, increase by 2 each round for 10 minutes.			
Squats	Legs, Glutes, Core	Lower hips below knees, keep chest up, push through heels to stand.			
Triceps Push-Ups	Triceps, Chest, Core	Hands under shoulders, keep elbows tight, lower chest to ground, push up.			
Mountain Climbers	Core, Cardio, Shoulders	Drive knees toward chest, keep core tight, move quickly.			
Workout No 151 (HIIT) – 20-Minute Tabata (20s Work, 10s Rest)		8 Rounds of 4 Exercises (20s on, 10s rest). Keep intensity high.			
Side Plank (Left)	Core, Obliques, Shoulders	Hold body in straight line, engage core, support weight on one forearm.			
Side Plank (Right)	Core, Obliques, Shoulders	Hold on opposite side, maintain stability, breathe evenly.			
Skater Squats	Legs, Glutes, Core	Balance on one leg, squat down, touch opposite hand to foot, alternate sides.			
Jumping Jacks	Cardio, Shoulders, Core	Jump feet apart while clapping hands overhead, then return to start.			
Workout No 152 (CrossFit) – 21-15-9 Reps Scheme		Perform 21 reps of each, then 15, then 9, as fast as possible.			
Burpees	Full Body, Cardio, Core	Drop into push-up, jump explosively, repeat.			
Reverse Crunch	Core, Lower Abs, Hip Flexors	Lift hips off floor, knees towards chest, control descent.			
Crab Toe Touch	Core, Shoulders, Coordination	In crab position, touch opposite hand to foot, alternate sides.			
Workout No 153 (HIIT) – Pyramid (10-8-6-4-2 Reps)		Start with 10 reps of each, decrease by 2 each round until you reach 2 reps.			
Inchworm	Core, Shoulders, Hamstrings	Walk hands forward to plank, hold, walk back to standing.			
Push-Up w/ Extension	Chest, Triceps, Core	Do a push-up, extend one arm forward, alternate sides.			
Tuck Jumps	Legs, Core, Cardio	Jump explosively, tuck knees to chest mid-air, land softly.			
Workout No 154 (CrossFit) – 12-Minute AMRAP		Complete as many rounds as possible in 12 minutes.			
10 Step-Ups	Legs, Glutes, Core	Step onto raised surface, alternate legs, keep controlled movement.			
12 Spiderman Push-Ups	Chest, Core, Shoulders	Lower into push-up while bringing knee to elbow, alternate sides.			
15 Donkey Kicks	Glutes, Core, Balance	On hands and knees, kick leg back and up, squeeze glutes.			

Workout	Main Muscle Groups	Instructions	Day 1	Day 2	Day 3
Workout No 155 (HIIT) – 5-Minute Burnout Finisher		Perform 5 exercises continuously for 1 minute each. No rest.			
High Knees	Cardio, Core, Legs	Drive knees high, move fast, pump arms.			
Squats	Legs, Glutes, Core	Lower hips below knees, keep chest up, push through heels.			
Plank	Core, Shoulders, Endurance	Hold plank position, engage core, maintain straight line.			
Mountain Climbers	Core, Cardio, Shoulders	Run in place from plank, drive knees toward chest.			
Jumping Jacks	Cardio, Shoulders, Core	Jump feet apart, clap hands overhead, return to start.			
Workout No 156 (CrossFit) – 12-Minute AMRAP (As Many Rounds As Possible)		Complete as many rounds as possible in 12 minutes. Keep a steady but intense pace.			
10 Burpees	Full Body, Core, Cardio	Jump, squat down, kick feet back into push-up, jump back up. Move quickly.			
15 Squats	Legs, Glutes, Core	Lower hips below knees, push through heels to rise. Keep chest up.			
20 Mountain Climbers	Core, Cardio, Shoulders	In plank, drive knees toward chest rapidly, keeping core engaged.			
Workout No 157 (HIIT) – 30 30 Intervals (5 Rounds)		30 seconds of work, 30 seconds of rest per exercise. Complete 5 rounds.			
Jumping Jacks	Cardio, Shoulders, Core	Jump feet apart while clapping hands overhead, then return to start. Keep high intensity.			
High Knees	Cardio, Core, Legs	Drive knees high, run in place fast, engage core and pump arms.			
Side-to-Side Push-Ups	Chest, Triceps, Core	Perform push-up, shift to one side, push up again, alternate sides.			
Bicycle Crunches	Core, Abs, Obliques	Lie on back, twist torso to bring elbow to opposite knee, extend opposite leg.			
Workout No 158 (CrossFit) – 5 Rounds for Time		Complete 5 rounds as fast as possible, keeping form strict. Rest only if needed.			
12 Box Jumps	Legs, Glutes, Cardio	Jump explosively onto a box, land softly, stand up fully, step down.			
10 Pike Push-Ups	Shoulders, Triceps, Core	In downward dog position, lower head toward ground, push up. Keep core engaged.			
15 Walking Lunges	Legs, Glutes, Core	Step forward into deep lunge, push through heel to stand, alternate legs.			
20 Flutter Kicks	Core, Lower Abs, Hip Flexors	Lie flat, keep legs straight, alternate kicking up and down. Keep lower back pressed down.			

Workout	Main Muscle Groups	Instructions	Day 1	Day 2	Day 3
Workout No 159 (HIIT) – 20-Minute Tabata (20s Work, 10s Rest, 8 Rounds Per Exercise)		Alternate between 2 exercises, doing 20 seconds of work followed by 10 seconds of rest. Repeat each pair for 8 rounds.			
Side Plank (Left)	Core, Obliques, Shoulders	Hold plank on one side, engage core, breathe steadily. Maintain a straight body line.			
Side Plank (Right)	Core, Obliques, Shoulders	Switch to opposite side and hold. Keep hips lifted, maintain steady breathing.			
Skater Squats	Legs, Glutes, Core	Balance on one leg, squat down, touch opposite hand to foot, then switch sides.			
Jumping Jacks	Cardio, Shoulders, Core	Jump feet apart, clap hands overhead, return to start. Keep pace fast.			
Workout No 160 (CrossFit) – 15-Minute Ladder (Increasing Reps Each Round)		Start with 2 reps per exercise, increase by 2 each round until 15 minutes are up.			
Squats	Legs, Glutes, Core	Lower hips below knees, drive through heels, keep chest up.			
Triceps Push-Ups	Triceps, Chest, Core	Hands under shoulders, elbows tight, lower chest to ground, push up.			
Mountain Climbers	Core, Cardio, Shoulders	Drive knees toward chest, keep core tight, move quickly.			
Workout No 161 (HIIT) – 10-Minute Burnout (No Rest, Max Effort)		Move continuously for 10 minutes, switching exercises every 45 seconds.			
Burpees	Full Body, Cardio, Core	Jump explosively, drop into push-up, jump back up, repeat continuously.			
Push-Backs	Shoulders, Arms, Core	From push-up position, push hips back toward heels, return to plank.			
Russian Twists	Core, Obliques, Abs	Sit with feet lifted, twist torso side to side, touch ground beside hips.			
Workout No 162 (CrossFit) – 21-15-9 Rep Scheme		Complete 21 reps of each, then 15, then 9, as fast as possible.			
Burpees	Full Body, Cardio, Core	Drop into a push-up, jump explosively, land softly, and repeat.			
Reverse Crunch	Core, Lower Abs, Hip Flexors	Lift hips off floor, knees towards chest, control descent.			
Crab Toe Touch	Core, Shoulders, Coordination	In crab position, touch opposite hand to foot, alternate sides.			
Workout No 163 (HIIT) – Pyramid (10-8-6-4-2 Reps)		Start with 10 reps of each, decrease by 2 each round until you reach 2 reps.			
Inchworm	Core, Shoulders, Hamstrings	Walk hands forward to plank, hold, walk back to standing.			
Push-Up w/ Extension	Chest, Triceps, Core	Perform push-up, extend one arm forward, alternate sides.			
Tuck Jumps	Legs, Core, Cardio	Jump explosively, tuck knees to chest mid-air, land softly.			

Workout	Main Muscle Groups	Instructions	Day 1	Day 2	Day 3
Workout No 164 (CrossFit) – 12-Minute AMRAP		Complete as many rounds as possible in 12 minutes.			
10 Step-Ups	Legs, Glutes, Core	Step onto raised surface, alternate legs, keep controlled movement.			
12 Spiderman Push-Ups	Chest, Core, Shoulders	Lower into push-up while bringing knee to elbow, alternate sides.			
15 Donkey Kicks	Glutes, Core, Balance	On hands and knees, kick leg back and up, squeeze glutes.			
Workout No 165 (HIIT) – 5-Minute Burnout Finisher		Perform 5 exercises continuously for 1 minute each. No rest.			
High Knees	Cardio, Core, Legs	Drive knees high, move fast, pump arms.			
Squats	Legs, Glutes, Core	Lower hips below knees, keep chest up, push through heels.			
Plank	Core, Shoulders, Endurance	Hold plank position, engage core, maintain straight line.			
Mountain Climbers	Core, Cardio, Shoulders	Run in place from plank, drive knees toward chest.			
Jumping Jacks	Cardio, Shoulders, Core	Jump feet apart, clap hands overhead, return to start.			
Workout No 166 (CrossFit) – 15-Minute AMRAP (As Many Rounds As Possible)		Complete as many rounds as possible in 15 minutes. Keep intensity high while maintaining proper form.			
10 Burpees	Full Body, Core, Cardio	Jump up, drop into a squat, kick feet back into push-up, jump back up explosively. Maintain steady rhythm and control.			
12 Squats	Legs, Glutes, Core	Stand shoulder-width apart, lower hips below knees, push through heels to rise. Keep chest up and core engaged.			
20 Mountain Climbers	Core, Cardio, Shoulders	In plank, drive knees toward chest quickly. Engage core throughout and move continuously.			
Workout No 167 (HIIT) – 30 30 Intervals (5 Rounds)		30 seconds of work, 30 seconds of rest per exercise. Complete 5 rounds.			
Jumping Jacks	Cardio, Shoulders, Core	Jump feet apart while clapping hands overhead, return to start. Keep pace high for maximum burn.			
High Knees	Cardio, Core, Legs	Drive knees high, run in place fast, engage core and pump arms aggressively.			
Side-to-Side Push-Ups	Chest, Triceps, Core	Perform a push-up, shift to one side, push up again. Alternate sides to engage core.			
Bicycle Crunches	Core, Abs, Obliques	Lie on back, twist torso to bring elbow to opposite knee, extend opposite leg straight.			

Workout	Main Muscle Groups	Instructions	Day 1	Day 2	Day 3
Workout No 168 (CrossFit) – 4 Rounds for Time		Complete 4 rounds as fast as possible. Rest only as needed.			
12 Box Jumps	Legs, Glutes, Cardio	Jump explosively onto a box, land softly, stand up fully, step down. Keep rhythm steady.			
10 Pike Push-Ups	Shoulders, Triceps, Core	In downward dog position, lower head toward ground, push up. Engage shoulders and arms.			
15 Walking Lunges	Legs, Glutes, Core	Step forward into deep lunge, push through heel to stand, alternate legs. Keep back upright.			
20 Flutter Kicks	Core, Lower Abs, Hip Flexors	Lie flat, keep legs straight, alternate kicking up and down. Keep lower back pressed down.			
Workout No 169 (HIIT) – 20-Minute Tabata (20s Work, 10s Rest, 8 Rounds Per Exercise)		Alternate between 2 exercises, doing 20 seconds of work followed by 10 seconds of rest. Repeat each pair for 8 rounds.			
Side Plank (Left)	Core, Obliques, Shoulders	Hold plank on one side, engage core, breathe steadily. Maintain a straight body line.			
Side Plank (Right)	Core, Obliques, Shoulders	Switch to opposite side and hold. Keep hips lifted, maintain steady breathing.			
Skater Squats	Legs, Glutes, Core	Balance on one leg, squat down, touch opposite hand to foot, then switch sides.			
Jumping Jacks	Cardio, Shoulders, Core	Jump feet apart, clap hands overhead, return to start. Keep pace fast and controlled.			
Workout No 170 (CrossFit) – 15-Minute Ladder (Increasing Reps Each Round)		Start with 2 reps per exercise, increase by 2 each round until 15 minutes are up.			
Squats	Legs, Glutes, Core	Lower hips below knees, drive through heels, keep chest up. Maintain a steady pace.			
Triceps Push-Ups	Triceps, Chest, Core	Hands under shoulders, elbows tight, lower chest to ground, push up. Keep form strict.			
Mountain Climbers	Core, Cardio, Shoulders	Drive knees toward chest, keep core tight, move quickly. Keep pace fast.			
Workout No 171 (HIIT) – 10-Minute Burnout (No Rest, Max Effort)		Move continuously for 10 minutes, switching exercises every 45 seconds.			
Burpees	Full Body, Cardio, Core	Jump explosively, drop into push-up, jump back up, repeat continuously. Keep intensity high.			
Push-Backs	Shoulders, Arms, Core	From push-up position, push hips back toward heels, return to plank. Engage core.			
Russian Twists	Core, Obliques, Abs	Sit with feet lifted, twist torso side to side, touch ground beside hips.			

Workout	Main Muscle Groups	Instructions	Day 1	Day 2	Day 3
Workout No 172 (CrossFit) – 21-15-9 Rep Scheme		Complete 21 reps of each, then 15, then 9, as fast as possible.			
Burpees	Full Body, Cardio, Core	Drop into a push-up, jump explosively, land softly, and repeat.			
Reverse Crunch	Core, Lower Abs, Hip Flexors	Lift hips off floor, knees towards chest, control descent. Keep core engaged.			
Crab Toe Touch	Core, Shoulders, Coordination	In crab position, touch opposite hand to foot, alternate sides. Maintain steady pace.			
Workout No 173 (HIIT) – Pyramid (10-8-6-4-2 Reps)		Start with 10 reps of each, decrease by 2 each round until you reach 2 reps.			
Inchworm	Core, Shoulders, Hamstrings	Walk hands forward to plank, hold, walk back to standing. Keep movements controlled.			
Push-Up w/ Extension	Chest, Triceps, Core	Perform push-up, extend one arm forward, alternate sides. Engage core.			
Tuck Jumps	Legs, Core, Cardio	Jump explosively, tuck knees to chest mid-air, land softly. Keep movements controlled.			
Workout No 174 (CrossFit) – 12-Minute AMRAP		Complete as many rounds as possible in 12 minutes.			
10 Step-Ups	Legs, Glutes, Core	Step onto raised surface, alternate legs, keep controlled movement.			
12 Spiderman Push-Ups	Chest, Core, Shoulders	Lower into push-up while bringing knee to elbow, alternate sides.			
15 Donkey Kicks	Glutes, Core, Balance	On hands and knees, kick leg back and up, squeeze glutes. Keep movements controlled.			
Workout No 175 (HIIT) – 5-Minute Burnout Finisher		Perform 5 exercises continuously for 1 minute each. No rest.			
High Knees	Cardio, Core, Legs	Drive knees high, move fast, pump arms aggressively.			
Squats	Legs, Glutes, Core	Lower hips below knees, keep chest up, push through heels. Maintain good posture.			
Plank	Core, Shoulders, Endurance	Hold plank position, engage core, maintain straight line. Keep breathing steady.			
Mountain Climbers	Core, Cardio, Shoulders	Run in place from plank, drive knees toward chest. Keep movements controlled.			
Workout No 176 (CrossFit) – 12-Minute AMRAP (As Many Rounds As Possible)		Complete as many rounds as possible in 12 minutes. Maintain intensity while keeping good form.			
10 Burpees	Full Body, Core, Cardio	Jump, drop into a squat, kick feet back into push-up, jump back up explosively.			
12 Squats	Legs, Glutes, Core	Stand shoulder-width apart, lower hips below knees, push through heels to rise.			
15 Mountain Climbers	Core, Cardio, Shoulders	In plank, drive knees toward chest quickly, keeping core engaged.			

Workout	Main Muscle Groups	Instructions	Day 1	Day 2	Day 3
Workout No 177 (HIIT) – 30 30 Intervals (4 Rounds)		30 seconds of work, 30 seconds of rest per exercise. Complete 4 rounds.			
Jumping Jacks	Cardio, Shoulders, Core	Jump feet apart while clapping hands overhead, return to start. Maintain high intensity.			
High Knees	Cardio, Core, Legs	Drive knees high, run in place fast, engage core and pump arms aggressively.			
Side-to-Side Push-Ups	Chest, Triceps, Core	Perform a push-up, shift to one side, push up again. Alternate sides to engage core.			
Bicycle Crunches	Core, Abs, Obliques	Lie on back, twist torso to bring elbow to opposite knee, extend opposite leg.			
Workout No 178 (CrossFit) – 4 Rounds for Time		Complete 4 rounds as fast as possible. Rest only as needed.			
12 Box Jumps	Legs, Glutes, Cardio	Jump explosively onto a box, land softly, stand up fully, step down.			
10 Pike Push-Ups	Shoulders, Triceps, Core	In downward dog position, lower head toward ground, push up. Keep core engaged.			
15 Walking Lunges	Legs, Glutes, Core	Step forward into a deep lunge, push through heel to stand, alternate legs.			
20 Flutter Kicks	Core, Lower Abs, Hip Flexors	Lie flat, keep legs straight, alternate kicking up and down. Keep lower back pressed down.			
Workout No 179 (HIIT) – 20-Minute Tabata (20s Work, 10s Rest, 8 Rounds Per Exercise)		Alternate between 2 exercises, doing 20 seconds of work followed by 10 seconds of rest. Repeat each pair for 8 rounds.			
Side Plank (Left)	Core, Obliques, Shoulders	Hold plank on one side, engage core, breathe steadily. Maintain a straight body line.			
Side Plank (Right)	Core, Obliques, Shoulders	Switch to opposite side and hold. Keep hips lifted, maintain steady breathing.			
Skater Squats	Legs, Glutes, Core	Balance on one leg, squat down, touch opposite hand to foot, then switch sides.			
Jumping Jacks	Cardio, Shoulders, Core	Jump feet apart, clap hands overhead, return to start. Keep pace fast and controlled.			
Workout No 180 (CrossFit) – 15-Minute Ladder (Increasing Reps Each Round)		Start with 2 reps per exercise, increase by 2 each round until 15 minutes are up.			
Squats	Legs, Glutes, Core	Lower hips below knees, drive through heels, keep chest up. Maintain a steady pace.			
Triceps Push-Ups	Triceps, Chest, Core	Hands under shoulders, elbows tight, lower chest to ground, push up. Keep form strict.			
Mountain Climbers	Core, Cardio, Shoulders	Drive knees toward chest, keep core tight, move quickly. Keep pace fast.			

	Workout	Main Muscle Groups	Instructions	Day 1	Day 2	Day 3
Workout No 181 (HIIT) – 10-Minute Burnout (No Rest, Max Effort)			Move continuously for 10 minutes, switching exercises every 45 seconds.			
Burpees		Full Body, Cardio, Core	Jump explosively, drop into push-up, jump back up, repeat continuously. Keep intensity high.			
Push-Backs		Shoulders, Arms, Core	From push-up position, push hips back toward heels, return to plank. Engage core.			
Russian Twists		Core, Obliques, Abs	Sit with feet lifted, twist torso side to side, touch ground beside hips.			
Workout No 182 (CrossFit) – 21-15-9 Rep Scheme			Complete 21 reps of each, then 15, then 9, as fast as possible.			
Burpees		Full Body, Cardio, Core	Drop into a push-up, jump explosively, land softly, and repeat.			
Reverse Crunch		Core, Lower Abs, Hip Flexors	Lift hips off floor, knees towards chest, control descent. Keep core engaged.			
Crab Toe Touch		Core, Shoulders, Coordination	In crab position, touch opposite hand to foot, alternate sides. Maintain steady pace.			
Workout No 183 (HIIT) – Pyramid (10-8-6-4-2 Reps)			Start with 10 reps of each, decrease by 2 each round until you reach 2 reps.			
Inchworm		Core, Shoulders, Hamstrings	Walk hands forward to plank, hold, walk back to standing. Keep movements controlled.			
Push-Up w/ Extension		Chest, Triceps, Core	Perform push-up, extend one arm forward, alternate sides. Engage core.			
Tuck Jumps		Legs, Core, Cardio	Jump explosively, tuck knees to chest mid-air, land softly. Keep movements controlled.			
Workout No 184 (CrossFit) – 12-Minute AMRAP			Complete as many rounds as possible in 12 minutes.			
10 Step-Ups		Legs, Glutes, Core	Step onto raised surface, alternate legs, keep controlled movement.			
12 Spiderman Push-Ups		Chest, Core, Shoulders	Lower into push-up while bringing knee to elbow, alternate sides.			
15 Donkey Kicks		Glutes, Core, Balance	On hands and knees, kick leg back and up, squeeze glutes. Keep movements controlled.			
Workout No 185 (HIIT) – 5-Minute Burnout Finisher			Perform 5 exercises continuously for 1 minute each. No rest.			
High Knees		Cardio, Core, Legs	Drive knees high, move fast, pump arms aggressively.			
Squats		Legs, Glutes, Core	Lower hips below knees, keep chest up, push through heels. Maintain good posture.			
Plank		Core, Shoulders, Endurance	Hold plank position, engage core, maintain straight line. Keep breathing steady.			
Mountain Climbers		Core, Cardio, Shoulders	Run in place from plank, drive knees toward chest. Keep movements controlled.			

	Workout	Main Muscle Groups	Instructions	Day 1	Day 2	Day 3
Workout No 186 (CrossFit) – 15-Minute AMRAP			Complete as many rounds as possible in 15 minutes. Maintain intensity and proper form.			
10 Burpees		Full Body, Core, Cardio	Jump, squat down, kick feet back into push-up, jump back up explosively.			
12 Squats		Legs, Glutes, Core	Stand shoulder-width apart, lower hips below knees, push through heels to rise.			
15 Mountain Climbers		Core, Cardio, Shoulders	In plank, drive knees toward chest quickly, keeping core engaged.			
Workout No 187 (HIIT) – 30 30 Intervals (4 Rounds)			30 seconds of work, 30 seconds of rest per exercise. Complete 4 rounds.			
Jumping Jacks		Cardio, Shoulders, Core	Jump feet apart while clapping hands overhead, return to start. Maintain high intensity.			
High Knees		Cardio, Core, Legs	Drive knees high, run in place fast, engage core and pump arms aggressively.			
Side-to-Side Push-Ups		Chest, Triceps, Core	Perform a push-up, shift to one side, push up again. Alternate sides to engage core.			
Bicycle Crunches		Core, Abs, Obliques	Lie on back, twist torso to bring elbow to opposite knee, extend opposite leg.			
Workout No 188 (CrossFit) – 4 Rounds for Time			Complete 4 rounds as fast as possible. Rest only as needed.			
12 Box Jumps		Legs, Glutes, Cardio	Jump explosively onto a box, land softly, stand up fully, step down.			
10 Pike Push-Ups		Shoulders, Triceps, Core	In downward dog position, lower head toward ground, push up. Keep core engaged.			
15 Walking Lunges		Legs, Glutes, Core	Step forward into a deep lunge, push through heel to stand, alternate legs.			
20 Flutter Kicks		Core, Lower Abs, Hip Flexors	Lie flat, keep legs straight, alternate kicking up and down. Keep lower back pressed down.			
Workout No 189 (HIIT) – 20-Minute Tabata (20s Work, 10s Rest, 8 Rounds Per Exercise)			Alternate between 2 exercises, doing 20 seconds of work followed by 10 seconds of rest. Repeat each pair for 8 rounds.			
Side Plank (Left)		Core, Obliques, Shoulders	Hold plank on one side, engage core, breathe steadily. Maintain a straight body line.			
Side Plank (Right)		Core, Obliques, Shoulders	Switch to opposite side and hold. Keep hips lifted, maintain steady breathing.			
Skater Squats		Legs, Glutes, Core	Balance on one leg, squat down, touch opposite hand to foot, then switch sides.			
Jumping Jacks		Cardio, Shoulders, Core	Jump feet apart, clap hands overhead, return to start. Keep pace fast and controlled.			

Workout	Main Muscle Groups	Instructions	Day 1	Day 2	Day 3
Workout No 190 (CrossFit) – 15-Minute Ladder (Increasing Reps Each Round)		Start with 2 reps per exercise, increase by 2 each round until 15 minutes are up.			
Squats	Legs, Glutes, Core	Lower hips below knees, drive through heels, keep chest up. Maintain a steady pace.			
Triceps Push-Ups	Triceps, Chest, Core	Hands under shoulders, elbows tight, lower chest to ground, push up. Keep form strict.			
Mountain Climbers	Core, Cardio, Shoulders	Drive knees toward chest, keep core tight, move quickly. Keep pace fast.			
Workout No 191 (HIIT) – 10-Minute Burnout (No Rest, Max Effort)		Move continuously for 10 minutes, switching exercises every 45 seconds.			
Burpees	Full Body, Cardio, Core	Jump explosively, drop into push-up, jump back up, repeat continuously. Keep intensity high.			
Push-Backs	Shoulders, Arms, Core	From push-up position, push hips back toward heels, return to plank. Engage core.			
Russian Twists	Core, Obliques, Abs	Sit with feet lifted, twist torso side to side, touch ground beside hips.			
Workout No 192 (CrossFit) – 21-15-9 Rep Scheme		Complete 21 reps of each, then 15, then 9, as fast as possible.			
Burpees	Full Body, Cardio, Core	Drop into a push-up, jump explosively, land softly, and repeat.			
Reverse Crunch	Core, Lower Abs, Hip Flexors	Lift hips off floor, knees towards chest, control descent. Keep core engaged.			
Crab Toe Touch	Core, Shoulders, Coordination	In crab position, touch opposite hand to foot, alternate sides. Maintain steady pace.			
Workout No 193 (HIIT) – Pyramid (10-8-6-4-2 Reps)		Start with 10 reps of each, decrease by 2 each round until you reach 2 reps.			
Inchworm	Core, Shoulders, Hamstrings	Walk hands forward to plank, hold, walk back to standing. Keep movements controlled.			
Push-Up w/ Extension	Chest, Triceps, Core	Perform push-up, extend one arm forward, alternate sides. Engage core.			
Tuck Jumps	Legs, Core, Cardio	Jump explosively, tuck knees to chest mid-air, land softly. Keep movements controlled.			
Workout No 194 (CrossFit) – 12-Minute AMRAP		Complete as many rounds as possible in 12 minutes.			
10 Step-Ups	Legs, Glutes, Core	Step onto raised surface, alternate legs, keep controlled movement.			
12 Spiderman Push-Ups	Chest, Core, Shoulders	Lower into push-up while bringing knee to elbow, alternate sides.			
15 Donkey Kicks	Glutes, Core, Balance	On hands and knees, kick leg back and up, squeeze glutes. Keep movements controlled.			

Workout	Main Muscle Groups	Instructions	Day 1	Day 2	Day 3
Workout No 195 (HIIT) – 5-Minute Burnout Finisher		Perform 5 exercises continuously for 1 minute each. No rest.			
High Knees	Cardio, Core, Legs	Drive knees high, move fast, pump arms aggressively.			
Squats	Legs, Glutes, Core	Lower hips below knees, keep chest up, push through heels. Maintain good posture.			
Plank	Core, Shoulders, Endurance	Hold plank position, engage core, maintain straight line. Keep breathing steady.			
Mountain Climbers	Core, Cardio, Shoulders	Run in place from plank, drive knees toward chest. Keep movements controlled.			
Workout No 196 (CrossFit) – 15-Minute AMRAP (As Many Rounds As Possible)		Complete as many rounds as possible in 15 minutes. Push hard while maintaining form.			
10 Burpees	Full Body, Core, Cardio	Jump, drop into a squat, kick feet back into push-up, jump back up explosively.			
15 Squats	Legs, Glutes, Core	Lower hips below knees, keep chest up, push through heels to rise.			
20 Mountain Climbers	Core, Cardio, Shoulders	In plank, drive knees toward chest rapidly, keeping core engaged.			
Workout No 197 (HIIT) – 30 30 Intervals (4 Rounds)		30 seconds of work, 30 seconds of rest per exercise. Complete 4 rounds.			
Jumping Jacks	Cardio, Shoulders, Core	Jump feet apart while clapping hands overhead, return to start. Keep high intensity.			
High Knees	Cardio, Core, Legs	Drive knees high, run in place fast, engage core and pump arms aggressively.			
Side-to-Side Push-Ups	Chest, Triceps, Core	Perform a push-up, shift to one side, push up again. Alternate sides to engage core.			
Bicycle Crunches	Core, Abs, Obliques	Lie on back, twist torso to bring elbow to opposite knee, extend opposite leg.			
Workout No 198 (CrossFit) – 4 Rounds for Time		Complete 4 rounds as fast as possible. Rest only as needed.			
12 Box Jumps	Legs, Glutes, Cardio	Jump explosively onto a box, land softly, stand up fully, step down.			
10 Pike Push-Ups	Shoulders, Triceps, Core	In downward dog position, lower head toward ground, push up. Keep core engaged.			
15 Walking Lunges	Legs, Glutes, Core	Step forward into deep lunge, push through heel to stand, alternate legs.			
20 Flutter Kicks	Core, Lower Abs, Hip Flexors	Lie flat, keep legs straight, alternate kicking up and down. Keep lower back pressed down.			

Workout	Main Muscle Groups	Instructions	Day 1	Day 2	Day 3
Workout No 199 (HIIT) – 20-Minute Tabata (20s Work, 10s Rest, 8 Rounds Per Exercise)		Alternate between 2 exercises, doing 20 seconds of work followed by 10 seconds of rest. Repeat each pair for 8 rounds.			
Side Plank (Left)	Core, Obliques, Shoulders	Hold plank on one side, engage core, breathe steadily. Maintain a straight body line.			
Side Plank (Right)	Core, Obliques, Shoulders	Switch to opposite side and hold. Keep hips lifted, maintain steady breathing.			
Skater Squats	Legs, Glutes, Core	Balance on one leg, squat down, touch opposite hand to foot, then switch sides.			
Jumping Jacks	Cardio, Shoulders, Core	Jump feet apart, clap hands overhead, return to start. Keep pace fast and controlled.			
Workout No 200 (CrossFit) – 15-Minute Ladder (Increasing Reps Each Round)		Start with 2 reps per exercise, increase by 2 each round until 15 minutes are up.			
Squats	Legs, Glutes, Core	Lower hips below knees, drive through heels, keep chest up. Maintain a steady pace.			
Triceps Push-Ups	Triceps, Chest, Core	Hands under shoulders, elbows tight, lower chest to ground, push up. Keep form strict.			
Mountain Climbers	Core, Cardio, Shoulders	Drive knees toward chest, keep core tight, move quickly. Keep pace fast.			
Workout No 201 (HIIT) – 10-Minute Burnout (No Rest, Max Effort)		Move continuously for 10 minutes, switching exercises every 45 seconds.			
Burpees	Full Body, Cardio, Core	Jump explosively, drop into push-up, jump back up, repeat continuously. Keep intensity high.			
Push-Backs	Shoulders, Arms, Core	From push-up position, push hips back toward heels, return to plank. Engage core.			
Russian Twists	Core, Obliques, Abs	Sit with feet lifted, twist torso side to side, touch ground beside hips.			
Workout No 202 (CrossFit) – 21-15-9 Rep Scheme		Complete 21 reps of each, then 15, then 9, as fast as possible.			
Burpees	Full Body, Cardio, Core	Drop into a push-up, jump explosively, land softly, and repeat.			
Reverse Crunch	Core, Lower Abs, Hip Flexors	Lift hips off floor, knees towards chest, control descent. Keep core engaged.			
Crab Toe Touch	Core, Shoulders, Coordination	In crab position, touch opposite hand to foot, alternate sides. Maintain steady pace.			

Workout	Main Muscle Groups	Instructions	Day 1	Day 2	Day 3
Workout No 203 (HIIT) – Pyramid (10-8-6-4-2 Reps)		Start with 10 reps of each, decrease by 2 each round until you reach 2 reps.			
Inchworm	Core, Shoulders, Hamstrings	Walk hands forward to plank, hold, walk back to standing. Keep movements controlled.			
Push-Up w/ Extension	Chest, Triceps, Core	Perform push-up, extend one arm forward, alternate sides. Engage core.			
Tuck Jumps	Legs, Core, Cardio	Jump explosively, tuck knees to chest mid-air, land softly. Keep movements controlled.			
Workout No 204 (CrossFit) – 12-Minute AMRAP		Complete as many rounds as possible in 12 minutes.			
10 Step-Ups	Legs, Glutes, Core	Step onto raised surface, alternate legs, keep controlled movement.			
12 Spiderman Push-Ups	Chest, Core, Shoulders	Lower into push-up while bringing knee to elbow, alternate sides.			
15 Donkey Kicks	Glutes, Core, Balance	On hands and knees, kick leg back and up, squeeze glutes. Keep movements controlled.			
Workout No 205 (HIIT) – 5-Minute Burnout Finisher		Perform 5 exercises continuously for 1 minute each. No rest.			
High Knees	Cardio, Core, Legs	Drive knees high, move fast, pump arms aggressively.			
Squats	Legs, Glutes, Core	Lower hips below knees, keep chest up, push through heels. Maintain good posture.			
Plank	Core, Shoulders, Endurance	Hold plank position, engage core, maintain straight line. Keep breathing steady.			
Mountain Climbers	Core, Cardio, Shoulders	Run in place from plank, drive knees toward chest. Keep movements controlled.			
Workout No 206 (CrossFit) – 15-Minute AMRAP (As Many Rounds As Possible)		Complete as many rounds as possible in 15 minutes. Keep moving at a high intensity.			
10 Burpees	Full Body, Core, Cardio	Jump, squat, kick feet back into push-up, return to standing, repeat. Move fast but maintain form.			
15 Squats	Legs, Glutes, Core	Lower hips below knees, push through heels to stand. Keep chest up.			
20 Mountain Climbers	Core, Cardio, Shoulders	In plank position, drive knees toward chest rapidly, maintaining a strong core.			

Workout	Main Muscle Groups	Instructions	Day 1	Day 2	Day 3
Workout No 207 (HIIT) – 30 30 Intervals (5 Rounds)		30 seconds of work, 30 seconds of rest per exercise. Complete 5 rounds.			
Jumping Jacks	Cardio, Shoulders, Core	Jump feet apart while clapping hands overhead, then return to start. Maintain a steady pace.			
High Knees	Cardio, Core, Legs	Drive knees high, run in place quickly, pump arms. Keep core engaged.			
Side-to-Side Push-Ups	Chest, Triceps, Core	Perform a push-up, shift to one side, push up again. Alternate sides.			
Bicycle Crunches	Core, Abs, Obliques	Lie on back, twist torso to bring elbow to opposite knee, extend opposite leg.			
Workout No 208 (CrossFit) – 4 Rounds for Time		Complete 4 rounds as fast as possible. Minimal rest.			
12 Box Jumps	Legs, Glutes, Cardio	Jump explosively onto a box, land softly, stand up fully, step down.			
10 Pike Push-Ups	Shoulders, Triceps, Core	In downward dog position, lower head toward ground, push up. Keep core tight.			
15 Walking Lunges	Legs, Glutes, Core	Step forward into a lunge, push through heel to stand, alternate legs.			
20 Flutter Kicks	Core, Lower Abs, Hip Flexors	Lie flat, keep legs straight, alternate kicking up and down. Maintain a strong core.			
Workout No 209 (HIIT) – 20-Minute Tabata (20s Work, 10s Rest, 8 Rounds Per Exercise)		Alternate between 2 exercises, 20s of work, 10s rest, 8 rounds per pair.			
Side Plank (Left)	Core, Obliques, Shoulders	Hold plank on one side, engage core, breathe steadily. Maintain straight posture.			
Side Plank (Right)	Core, Obliques, Shoulders	Switch sides and hold plank. Keep hips lifted, maintain steady breathing.			
Skater Squats	Legs, Glutes, Core	Balance on one leg, squat down, touch opposite hand to foot, switch sides.			
Jumping Jacks	Cardio, Shoulders, Core	Jump feet apart, clap hands overhead, return to start. Keep steady rhythm.			
Workout No 210 (CrossFit) – 15-Minute Ladder (Increasing Reps Each Round)		Start with 2 reps per exercise, increase by 2 each round until 15 minutes are up.			
Squats	Legs, Glutes, Core	Lower hips below knees, drive through heels, keep chest up.			
Triceps Push-Ups	Triceps, Chest, Core	Hands under shoulders, elbows tight, lower chest to ground, push up.			
Mountain Climbers	Core, Cardio, Shoulders	Drive knees toward chest, keep core tight, move quickly.			

	Workout	Main Muscle Groups	Instructions	Day 1	Day 2	Day 3
Workout No 211 (HIIT) – 10-Minute Burnout (No Rest, Max Effort)			Move continuously for 10 minutes, switching exercises every 45 seconds.			
Burpees		Full Body, Cardio, Core	Jump explosively, drop into push-up, jump back up, repeat continuously.			
Push-Backs		Shoulders, Arms, Core	From push-up position, push hips back toward heels, return to plank.			
Russian Twists		Core, Obliques, Abs	Sit with feet lifted, twist torso side to side, touch ground beside hips.			
Workout No 212 (CrossFit) – 21-15-9 Rep Scheme			Complete 21 reps of each, then 15, then 9, as fast as possible.			
Burpees		Full Body, Cardio, Core	Drop into a push-up, jump explosively, land softly, and repeat.			
Reverse Crunch		Core, Lower Abs, Hip Flexors	Lift hips off floor, knees towards chest, control descent. Keep core engaged.			
Crab Toe Touch		Core, Shoulders, Coordination	In crab position, touch opposite hand to foot, alternate sides.			
Workout No 213 (HIIT) – Pyramid (10-8-6-4-2 Reps)			Start with 10 reps of each, decrease by 2 each round until you reach 2 reps.			
Inchworm		Core, Shoulders, Hamstrings	Walk hands forward to plank, hold, walk back to standing. Keep movements controlled.			
Push-Up w/ Extension		Chest, Triceps, Core	Perform push-up, extend one arm forward, alternate sides. Engage core.			
Tuck Jumps		Legs, Core, Cardio	Jump explosively, tuck knees to chest mid-air, land softly.			
Workout No 214 (CrossFit) – 12-Minute AMRAP			Complete as many rounds as possible in 12 minutes.			
10 Step-Ups		Legs, Glutes, Core	Step onto raised surface, alternate legs, keep controlled movement.			
12 Spiderman Push-Ups		Chest, Core, Shoulders	Lower into push-up while bringing knee to elbow, alternate sides.			
15 Donkey Kicks		Glutes, Core, Balance	On hands and knees, kick leg back and up, squeeze glutes.			
Workout No 215 (HIIT) – 5-Minute Burnout Finisher			Perform 5 exercises continuously for 1 minute each. No rest.			
High Knees		Cardio, Core, Legs	Drive knees high, move fast, pump arms aggressively.			
Squats		Legs, Glutes, Core	Lower hips below knees, keep chest up, push through heels.			
Plank		Core, Shoulders, Endurance	Hold plank position, engage core, maintain straight line.			
Mountain Climbers		Core, Cardio, Shoulders	Run in place from plank, drive knees toward chest.			

Workout	Main Muscle Groups	Instructions	Day 1	Day 2	Day 3
Workout No 216 (CrossFit) – 12-Minute AMRAP (As Many Rounds As Possible)		Complete as many rounds as possible in 12 minutes, keeping a consistent pace.			
10 Burpees	Full Body, Core, Cardio	Jump, squat down, kick feet back into push-up, jump back up explosively.			
15 Squats	Legs, Glutes, Core	Stand shoulder-width apart, lower hips below knees, push through heels to rise.			
20 Mountain Climbers	Core, Cardio, Shoulders	In plank, drive knees toward chest quickly, keeping core engaged.			
Workout No 217 (HIIT) – 30 30 Intervals (5 Rounds)		30 seconds of work, 30 seconds of rest per exercise. Complete 5 rounds.			
Jumping Jacks	Cardio, Shoulders, Core	Jump feet apart while clapping hands overhead, return to start. Maintain high intensity.			
High Knees	Cardio, Core, Legs	Drive knees high, run in place fast, engage core and pump arms aggressively.			
Side-to-Side Push-Ups	Chest, Triceps, Core	Perform a push-up, shift to one side, push up again. Alternate sides to engage core.			
Bicycle Crunches	Core, Abs, Obliques	Lie on back, twist torso to bring elbow to opposite knee, extend opposite leg.			
Workout No 218 (CrossFit) – 4 Rounds for Time		Complete 4 rounds as fast as possible. Rest only as needed.			
12 Box Jumps	Legs, Glutes, Cardio	Jump explosively onto a box, land softly, stand up fully, step down.			
10 Pike Push-Ups	Shoulders, Triceps, Core	In downward dog position, lower head toward ground, push up. Keep core engaged.			
15 Walking Lunges	Legs, Glutes, Core	Step forward into a deep lunge, push through heel to stand, alternate legs.			
20 Flutter Kicks	Core, Lower Abs, Hip Flexors	Lie flat, keep legs straight, alternate kicking up and down. Keep lower back pressed down.			
Workout No 219 (HIIT) – 20-Minute Tabata (20s Work, 10s Rest, 8 Rounds Per Exercise)		Alternate between 2 exercises, doing 20 seconds of work followed by 10 seconds of rest. Repeat each pair for 8 rounds.			
Side Plank (Left)	Core, Obliques, Shoulders	Hold plank on one side, engage core, breathe steadily. Maintain a straight body line.			
Side Plank (Right)	Core, Obliques, Shoulders	Switch to opposite side and hold. Keep hips lifted, maintain steady breathing.			
Skater Squats	Legs, Glutes, Core	Balance on one leg, squat down, touch opposite hand to foot, then switch sides.			
Jumping Jacks	Cardio, Shoulders, Core	Jump feet apart, clap hands overhead, return to start. Keep pace fast and controlled.			

Workout	Main Muscle Groups	Instructions	Day 1	Day 2	Day 3
Workout No 220 (CrossFit) – 15-Minute Ladder (Increasing Reps Each Round)		Start with 2 reps per exercise, increase by 2 each round until 15 minutes are up.			
Squats	Legs, Glutes, Core	Lower hips below knees, drive through heels, keep chest up. Maintain a steady pace.			
Triceps Push-Ups	Triceps, Chest, Core	Hands under shoulders, elbows tight, lower chest to ground, push up. Keep form strict.			
Mountain Climbers	Core, Cardio, Shoulders	Drive knees toward chest, keep core tight, move quickly. Keep pace fast.			
Workout No 221 (HIIT) – 10-Minute Burnout (No Rest, Max Effort)		Move continuously for 10 minutes, switching exercises every 45 seconds.			
Burpees	Full Body, Cardio, Core	Jump explosively, drop into push-up, jump back up, repeat continuously. Keep intensity high.			
Push-Backs	Shoulders, Arms, Core	From push-up position, push hips back toward heels, return to plank. Engage core.			
Russian Twists	Core, Obliques, Abs	Sit with feet lifted, twist torso side to side, touch ground beside hips.			
Workout No 222 (CrossFit) – 21-15-9 Rep Scheme		Complete 21 reps of each, then 15, then 9, as fast as possible.			
Burpees	Full Body, Cardio, Core	Drop into a push-up, jump explosively, land softly, and repeat.			
Reverse Crunch	Core, Lower Abs, Hip Flexors	Lift hips off floor, knees towards chest, control descent. Keep core engaged.			
Crab Toe Touch	Core, Shoulders, Coordination	In crab position, touch opposite hand to foot, alternate sides. Maintain steady pace.			
Workout No 223 (HIIT) – Pyramid (10-8-6-4-2 Reps)		Start with 10 reps of each, decrease by 2 each round until you reach 2 reps.			
Inchworm	Core, Shoulders, Hamstrings	Walk hands forward to plank, hold, walk back to standing. Keep movements controlled.			
Push-Up w/ Extension	Chest, Triceps, Core	Perform push-up, extend one arm forward, alternate sides. Engage core.			
Tuck Jumps	Legs, Core, Cardio	Jump explosively, tuck knees to chest mid-air, land softly. Keep movements controlled.			
Workout No 224 (CrossFit) – 12-Minute AMRAP		Complete as many rounds as possible in 12 minutes.			
10 Step-Ups	Legs, Glutes, Core	Step onto raised surface, alternate legs, keep controlled movement.			
12 Spiderman Push-Ups	Chest, Core, Shoulders	Lower into push-up while bringing knee to elbow, alternate sides.			
15 Donkey Kicks	Glutes, Core, Balance	On hands and knees, kick leg back and up, squeeze glutes. Keep movements controlled.			

	Workout	Main Muscle Groups	Instructions	Day 1	Day 2	Day 3
Workout No 225 (HIIT) – 5-Minute Burnout Finisher			Perform 5 exercises continuously for 1 minute each. No rest.			
High Knees		Cardio, Core, Legs	Drive knees high, move fast, pump arms aggressively.			
Squats		Legs, Glutes, Core	Lower hips below knees, keep chest up, push through heels. Maintain good posture.			
Plank		Core, Shoulders, Endurance	Hold plank position, engage core, maintain straight line. Keep breathing steady.			
Mountain Climbers		Core, Cardio, Shoulders	Run in place from plank, drive knees toward chest. Keep movements controlled.			
Workout No 226 (CrossFit) – 15-Minute AMRAP (As Many Rounds As Possible)			Complete as many rounds as possible in 15 minutes. Push hard while maintaining form.			
10 Burpees		Full Body, Core, Cardio	Jump, drop into a squat, kick feet back into push-up, jump back up explosively.			
15 Squats		Legs, Glutes, Core	Lower hips below knees, keep chest up, push through heels to rise.			
20 Mountain Climbers		Core, Cardio, Shoulders	In plank, drive knees toward chest rapidly, keeping core engaged.			
Workout No 227 (HIIT) – 30 30 Intervals (4 Rounds)			30 seconds of work, 30 seconds of rest per exercise. Complete 4 rounds.			
Jumping Jacks		Cardio, Shoulders, Core	Jump feet apart while clapping hands overhead, return to start. Keep high intensity.			
High Knees		Cardio, Core, Legs	Drive knees high, run in place fast, engage core and pump arms aggressively.			
Side-to-Side Push-Ups		Chest, Triceps, Core	Perform a push-up, shift to one side, push up again. Alternate sides to engage core.			
Bicycle Crunches		Core, Abs, Obliques	Lie on back, twist torso to bring elbow to opposite knee, extend opposite leg.			
Workout No 228 (CrossFit) – 4 Rounds for Time			Complete 4 rounds as fast as possible. Rest only as needed.			
12 Box Jumps		Legs, Glutes, Cardio	Jump explosively onto a box, land softly, stand up fully, step down.			
10 Pike Push-Ups		Shoulders, Triceps, Core	In downward dog position, lower head toward ground, push up. Keep core engaged.			
15 Walking Lunges		Legs, Glutes, Core	Step forward into deep lunge, push through heel to stand, alternate legs.			
20 Flutter Kicks		Core, Lower Abs, Hip Flexors	Lie flat, keep legs straight, alternate kicking up and down. Keep lower back pressed down.			

Workout	Main Muscle Groups	Instructions	Day 1	Day 2	Day 3
Workout No 229 (HIIT) – 20-Minute Tabata (20s Work, 10s Rest, 8 Rounds Per Exercise)		Alternate between 2 exercises, doing 20 seconds of work followed by 10 seconds of rest. Repeat each pair for 8 rounds.			
Side Plank (Left)	Core, Obliques, Shoulders	Hold plank on one side, engage core, breathe steadily. Maintain a straight body line.			
Side Plank (Right)	Core, Obliques, Shoulders	Switch to opposite side and hold. Keep hips lifted, maintain steady breathing.			
Skater Squats	Legs, Glutes, Core	Balance on one leg, squat down, touch opposite hand to foot, then switch sides.			
Jumping Jacks	Cardio, Shoulders, Core	Jump feet apart, clap hands overhead, return to start. Keep pace fast and controlled.			
Workout No 230 (CrossFit) – 15-Minute Ladder (Increasing Reps Each Round)		Start with 2 reps per exercise, increase by 2 each round until 15 minutes are up.			
Squats	Legs, Glutes, Core	Lower hips below knees, drive through heels, keep chest up. Maintain a steady pace.			
Triceps Push-Ups	Triceps, Chest, Core	Hands under shoulders, elbows tight, lower chest to ground, push up. Keep form strict.			
Mountain Climbers	Core, Cardio, Shoulders	Drive knees toward chest, keep core tight, move quickly. Keep pace fast.			
Workout No 231 (HIIT) – 10-Minute Burnout (No Rest, Max Effort)		Move continuously for 10 minutes, switching exercises every 45 seconds.			
Burpees	Full Body, Cardio, Core	Jump explosively, drop into push-up, jump back up, repeat continuously. Keep intensity high.			
Push-Backs	Shoulders, Arms, Core	From push-up position, push hips back toward heels, return to plank. Engage core.			
Russian Twists	Core, Obliques, Abs	Sit with feet lifted, twist torso side to side, touch ground beside hips.			
Workout No 232 (CrossFit) – 21-15-9 Rep Scheme		Complete 21 reps of each, then 15, then 9, as fast as possible.			
Burpees	Full Body, Cardio, Core	Drop into a push-up, jump explosively, land softly, and repeat.			
Reverse Crunch	Core, Lower Abs, Hip Flexors	Lift hips off floor, knees towards chest, control descent. Keep core engaged.			
Crab Toe Touch	Core, Shoulders, Coordination	In crab position, touch opposite hand to foot, alternate sides. Maintain steady pace.			

Workout	Main Muscle Groups	Instructions	Day 1	Day 2	Day 3
Workout No 233 (HIIT) – Pyramid (10-8-6-4-2 Reps)		Start with 10 reps of each, decrease by 2 each round until you reach 2 reps.			
Inchworm	Core, Shoulders, Hamstrings	Walk hands forward to plank, hold, walk back to standing. Keep movements controlled.			
Push-Up w/ Extension	Chest, Triceps, Core	Perform push-up, extend one arm forward, alternate sides. Engage core.			
Tuck Jumps	Legs, Core, Cardio	Jump explosively, tuck knees to chest mid-air, land softly. Keep movements controlled.			
Workout No 234 (CrossFit) – 12-Minute AMRAP		Complete as many rounds as possible in 12 minutes.			
10 Step-Ups	Legs, Glutes, Core	Step onto raised surface, alternate legs, keep controlled movement.			
12 Spiderman Push-Ups	Chest, Core, Shoulders	Lower into push-up while bringing knee to elbow, alternate sides.			
15 Donkey Kicks	Glutes, Core, Balance	On hands and knees, kick leg back and up, squeeze glutes. Keep movements controlled.			
Workout No 235 (HIIT) – 5-Minute Burnout Finisher		Perform 5 exercises continuously for 1 minute each. No rest.			
High Knees	Cardio, Core, Legs	Drive knees high, move fast, pump arms aggressively.			
Squats	Legs, Glutes, Core	Lower hips below knees, keep chest up, push through heels. Maintain good posture.			
Plank	Core, Shoulders, Endurance	Hold plank position, engage core, maintain straight line. Keep breathing steady.			
Mountain Climbers	Core, Cardio, Shoulders	Run in place from plank, drive knees toward chest. Keep movements controlled.			
Workout No 236 (CrossFit) – 12-Minute AMRAP (As Many Rounds As Possible)		Complete as many rounds as possible in 12 minutes. Move fast, keep good form.			
10 Burpees	Full Body, Core, Cardio	Jump, drop into push-up, jump back up. Keep intensity high and land softly.			
15 Squats	Legs, Glutes, Core	Lower hips below knees, push through heels to rise, keep chest up.			
20 Mountain Climbers	Core, Cardio, Shoulders	In plank, drive knees toward chest, move quickly but controlled.			
Workout No 237 (HIIT) – 30 30 Intervals (4 Rounds)		30 seconds of work, 30 seconds rest per exercise. 4 total rounds.			
Jumping Jacks	Cardio, Shoulders, Core	Jump feet apart while clapping hands overhead, return to start. Move fast.			
High Knees	Cardio, Core, Legs	Run in place, drive knees high, pump arms aggressively.			
Side-to-Side Push-Ups	Chest, Triceps, Core	Do a push-up, shift to one side, push up again. Switch sides.			
Bicycle Crunches	Core, Abs, Obliques	Lie back, twist torso, bring elbow to opposite knee, extend leg.			

Workout	Main Muscle Groups	Instructions	Day 1	Day 2	Day 3
Workout No 238 (CrossFit) – 4 Rounds for Time		Complete 4 rounds as fast as possible. Minimal rest.			
12 Box Jumps	Legs, Glutes, Cardio	Jump onto a box, land softly, step down. Keep core tight.			
10 Pike Push-Ups	Shoulders, Triceps, Core	From downward dog position, lower head to ground, push up.			
15 Walking Lunges	Legs, Glutes, Core	Step into deep lunge, push through heel to stand, alternate legs.			
20 Flutter Kicks	Core, Lower Abs, Hip Flexors	Lie flat, keep legs straight, alternate kicking up and down.			
Workout No 239 (HIIT) – 20-Minute Tabata (20s Work, 10s Rest, 8 Rounds Per Exercise)		Alternate between 2 exercises, 20 seconds work, 10 seconds rest. 8 rounds.			
Side Plank (Left)	Core, Obliques, Shoulders	Hold plank on one side, engage core, breathe steadily. Stay straight.			
Side Plank (Right)	Core, Obliques, Shoulders	Switch sides, keep hips lifted, core tight. Breathe evenly.			
Skater Squats	Legs, Glutes, Core	Balance on one leg, squat, touch opposite hand to foot, switch sides.			
Jumping Jacks	Cardio, Shoulders, Core	Jump feet apart, clap hands overhead, return to start. Maintain rhythm.			
Workout No 240 (CrossFit) – 15-Minute Ladder (Increasing Reps Each Round)		Start with 2 reps per exercise, increase by 2 each round until 15 minutes are up.			
Squats	Legs, Glutes, Core	Lower hips below knees, drive through heels, keep chest up.			
Triceps Push-Ups	Triceps, Chest, Core	Hands under shoulders, elbows tight, lower chest to ground, push up.			
Mountain Climbers	Core, Cardio, Shoulders	Drive knees toward chest, keep core tight, move fast.			
Workout No 241 (HIIT) – 10-Minute Burnout (No Rest, Max Effort)		Move continuously for 10 minutes, switch exercises every 45 seconds.			
Burpees	Full Body, Cardio, Core	Jump explosively, drop into push-up, jump back up, repeat.			
Push-Backs	Shoulders, Arms, Core	From push-up position, push hips back toward heels, return to plank.			
Russian Twists	Core, Obliques, Abs	Sit with feet lifted, twist torso side to side, touch ground beside hips.			
Workout No 242 (CrossFit) – 21-15-9 Rep Scheme		Complete 21 reps of each, then 15, then 9, as fast as possible.			
Burpees	Full Body, Cardio, Core	Drop into push-up, jump explosively, land softly, repeat.			
Reverse Crunch	Core, Lower Abs, Hip Flexors	Lift hips off floor, knees toward chest, control descent.			
Crab Toe Touch	Core, Shoulders, Coordination	In crab position, touch opposite hand to foot, switch sides.			

Workout	Main Muscle Groups	Instructions	Day 1	Day 2	Day 3
Workout No 243 (HIIT) – Pyramid (10-8-6-4-2 Reps)		Start with 10 reps of each, decrease by 2 each round until 2 reps.			
Inchworm	Core, Shoulders, Hamstrings	Walk hands forward to plank, hold, walk back to standing.			
Push-Up w/ Extension	Chest, Triceps, Core	Do push-up, extend one arm forward, alternate sides.			
Tuck Jumps	Legs, Core, Cardio	Jump explosively, tuck knees to chest mid-air, land softly.			
Workout No 244 (CrossFit) – 12-Minute AMRAP		Complete as many rounds as possible in 12 minutes.			
10 Step-Ups	Legs, Glutes, Core	Step onto raised surface, alternate legs, keep controlled movement.			
12 Spiderman Push-Ups	Chest, Core, Shoulders	Lower into push-up while bringing knee to elbow, alternate sides.			
15 Donkey Kicks	Glutes, Core, Balance	On hands and knees, kick leg back and up, squeeze glutes.			
Workout No 245 (HIIT) – 5-Minute Burnout Finisher		Perform 5 exercises continuously for 1 minute each. No rest.			
High Knees	Cardio, Core, Legs	Drive knees high, move fast, pump arms aggressively.			
Squats	Legs, Glutes, Core	Lower hips below knees, keep chest up, push through heels.			
Plank	Core, Shoulders, Endurance	Hold plank position, engage core, maintain straight line.			
Mountain Climbers	Core, Cardio, Shoulders	Run in place from plank, drive knees toward chest.			
Workout No 246 (CrossFit) – 15-Minute AMRAP (As Many Rounds As Possible)		Complete as many rounds as possible in 15 minutes. Move fast, maintain proper form.			
10 Burpees	Full Body, Core, Cardio	Jump, drop into push-up, jump back up. Keep intensity high and land softly.			
15 Squats	Legs, Glutes, Core	Lower hips below knees, push through heels to rise, keep chest up.			
20 Mountain Climbers	Core, Cardio, Shoulders	In plank, drive knees toward chest, move quickly but controlled.			
Workout No 247 (HIIT) – 30 30 Intervals (4 Rounds)		30 seconds of work, 30 seconds rest per exercise. 4 total rounds.			
Jumping Jacks	Cardio, Shoulders, Core	Jump feet apart while clapping hands overhead, return to start. Move fast.			
High Knees	Cardio, Core, Legs	Run in place, drive knees high, pump arms aggressively.			
Side-to-Side Push-Ups	Chest, Triceps, Core	Do a push-up, shift to one side, push up again. Switch sides.			
Bicycle Crunches	Core, Abs, Obliques	Lie back, twist torso, bring elbow to opposite knee, extend leg.			

Workout	Main Muscle Groups	Instructions	Day 1	Day 2	Day 3
Workout No 248 (CrossFit) – 4 Rounds for Time		Complete 4 rounds as fast as possible. Minimal rest.			
12 Box Jumps	Legs, Glutes, Cardio	Jump onto a box, land softly, step down. Keep core tight.			
10 Pike Push-Ups	Shoulders, Triceps, Core	From downward dog position, lower head to ground, push up.			
15 Walking Lunges	Legs, Glutes, Core	Step into deep lunge, push through heel to stand, alternate legs.			
20 Flutter Kicks	Core, Lower Abs, Hip Flexors	Lie flat, keep legs straight, alternate kicking up and down.			
Workout No 249 (HIIT) – 20-Minute Tabata (20s Work, 10s Rest, 8 Rounds Per Exercise)		Alternate between 2 exercises, 20 seconds work, 10 seconds rest. 8 rounds.			
Side Plank (Left)	Core, Obliques, Shoulders	Hold plank on one side, engage core, breathe steadily. Stay straight.			
Side Plank (Right)	Core, Obliques, Shoulders	Switch sides, keep hips lifted, core tight. Breathe evenly.			
Skater Squats	Legs, Glutes, Core	Balance on one leg, squat, touch opposite hand to foot, switch sides.			
Jumping Jacks	Cardio, Shoulders, Core	Jump feet apart, clap hands overhead, return to start. Maintain rhythm.			
Workout No 250 (CrossFit) – 15-Minute Ladder (Increasing Reps Each Round)		Start with 2 reps per exercise, increase by 2 each round until 15 minutes are up.			
Squats	Legs, Glutes, Core	Lower hips below knees, drive through heels, keep chest up.			
Triceps Push-Ups	Triceps, Chest, Core	Hands under shoulders, elbows tight, lower chest to ground, push up.			
Mountain Climbers	Core, Cardio, Shoulders	Drive knees toward chest, keep core tight, move fast.			
Workout No 251 (HIIT) – 10-Minute Burnout (No Rest, Max Effort)		Move continuously for 10 minutes, switch exercises every 45 seconds.			
Burpees	Full Body, Cardio, Core	Jump explosively, drop into push-up, jump back up, repeat.			
Push-Backs	Shoulders, Arms, Core	From push-up position, push hips back toward heels, return to plank.			
Russian Twists	Core, Obliques, Abs	Sit with feet lifted, twist torso side to side, touch ground beside hips.			
Workout No 252 (CrossFit) – 21-15-9 Rep Scheme		Complete 21 reps of each, then 15, then 9, as fast as possible.			
Burpees	Full Body, Cardio, Core	Drop into push-up, jump explosively, land softly, repeat.			
Reverse Crunch	Core, Lower Abs, Hip Flexors	Lift hips off floor, knees toward chest, control descent.			
Crab Toe Touch	Core, Shoulders, Coordination	In crab position, touch opposite hand to foot, switch sides.			

Workout	Main Muscle Groups	Instructions	Day 1	Day 2	Day 3
Workout No 253 (HIIT) – Pyramid (10-8-6-4-2 Reps)		Start with 10 reps of each, decrease by 2 each round until 2 reps.			
Inchworm	Core, Shoulders, Hamstrings	Walk hands forward to plank, hold, walk back to standing.			
Push-Up w/ Extension	Chest, Triceps, Core	Do push-up, extend one arm forward, alternate sides.			
Tuck Jumps	Legs, Core, Cardio	Jump explosively, tuck knees to chest mid-air, land softly.			
Workout No 254 (CrossFit) – 12-Minute AMRAP		Complete as many rounds as possible in 12 minutes.			
10 Step-Ups	Legs, Glutes, Core	Step onto raised surface, alternate legs, keep controlled movement.			
12 Spiderman Push-Ups	Chest, Core, Shoulders	Lower into push-up while bringing knee to elbow, alternate sides.			
15 Donkey Kicks	Glutes, Core, Balance	On hands and knees, kick leg back and up, squeeze glutes.			
Workout No 255 (HIIT) – 5-Minute Burnout Finisher		Perform 5 exercises continuously for 1 minute each. No rest.			
High Knees	Cardio, Core, Legs	Drive knees high, move fast, pump arms aggressively.			
Squats	Legs, Glutes, Core	Lower hips below knees, keep chest up, push through heels.			
Plank	Core, Shoulders, Endurance	Hold plank position, engage core, maintain straight line.			
Mountain Climbers	Core, Cardio, Shoulders	Run in place from plank, drive knees toward chest.			
Workout No 256 (CrossFit) – 12-Minute AMRAP (As Many Rounds As Possible)		Complete as many rounds as possible in 12 minutes. Move fast while maintaining good form.			
10 Burpees	Full Body, Core, Cardio	Jump, drop into a push-up, jump back up. Move fast and land softly.			
15 Squats	Legs, Glutes, Core	Lower hips below knees, push through heels to rise, keep chest up.			
20 Mountain Climbers	Core, Cardio, Shoulders	In plank, drive knees toward chest, move quickly but controlled.			
Workout No 257 (HIIT) – 30 30 Intervals (4 Rounds)		30 seconds of work, 30 seconds rest per exercise. 4 total rounds.			
Jumping Jacks	Cardio, Shoulders, Core	Jump feet apart while clapping hands overhead, return to start. Move fast.			
High Knees	Cardio, Core, Legs	Run in place, drive knees high, pump arms aggressively.			
Side-to-Side Push-Ups	Chest, Triceps, Core	Do a push-up, shift to one side, push up again. Switch sides.			
Bicycle Crunches	Core, Abs, Obliques	Lie back, twist torso, bring elbow to opposite knee, extend leg.			

Workout	Main Muscle Groups	Instructions	Day 1	Day 2	Day 3
Workout No 258 (CrossFit) – 4 Rounds for Time		Complete 4 rounds as fast as possible. Minimal rest.			
12 Box Jumps	Legs, Glutes, Cardio	Jump onto a box, land softly, step down. Keep core tight.			
10 Pike Push-Ups	Shoulders, Triceps, Core	From downward dog position, lower head to ground, push up.			
15 Walking Lunges	Legs, Glutes, Core	Step into deep lunge, push through heel to stand, alternate legs.			
20 Flutter Kicks	Core, Lower Abs, Hip Flexors	Lie flat, keep legs straight, alternate kicking up and down.			
Workout No 259 (HIIT) – 20-Minute Tabata (20s Work, 10s Rest, 8 Rounds Per Exercise)		Alternate between 2 exercises, 20 seconds work, 10 seconds rest. 8 rounds.			
Side Plank (Left)	Core, Obliques, Shoulders	Hold plank on one side, engage core, breathe steadily. Stay straight.			
Side Plank (Right)	Core, Obliques, Shoulders	Switch sides, keep hips lifted, core tight. Breathe evenly.			
Skater Squats	Legs, Glutes, Core	Balance on one leg, squat, touch opposite hand to foot, switch sides.			
Jumping Jacks	Cardio, Shoulders, Core	Jump feet apart, clap hands overhead, return to start. Maintain rhythm.			
Workout No 260 (CrossFit) – 15-Minute Ladder (Increasing Reps Each Round)		Start with 2 reps per exercise, increase by 2 each round until 15 minutes are up.			
Squats	Legs, Glutes, Core	Lower hips below knees, drive through heels, keep chest up.			
Triceps Push-Ups	Triceps, Chest, Core	Hands under shoulders, elbows tight, lower chest to ground, push up.			
Mountain Climbers	Core, Cardio, Shoulders	Drive knees toward chest, keep core tight, move fast.			
Workout No 261 (HIIT) – 10-Minute Burnout (No Rest, Max Effort)		Move continuously for 10 minutes, switch exercises every 45 seconds.			
Burpees	Full Body, Cardio, Core	Jump explosively, drop into push-up, jump back up, repeat.			
Push-Backs	Shoulders, Arms, Core	From push-up position, push hips back toward heels, return to plank.			
Russian Twists	Core, Obliques, Abs	Sit with feet lifted, twist torso side to side, touch ground beside hips.			
Workout No 262 (CrossFit) – 21-15-9 Rep Scheme		Complete 21 reps of each, then 15, then 9, as fast as possible.			
Burpees	Full Body, Cardio, Core	Drop into push-up, jump explosively, land softly, repeat.			
Reverse Crunch	Core, Lower Abs, Hip Flexors	Lift hips off floor, knees toward chest, control descent.			
Crab Toe Touch	Core, Shoulders, Coordination	In crab position, touch opposite hand to foot, switch sides.			

Workout	Main Muscle Groups	Instructions	Day 1	Day 2	Day 3
Workout No 263 (HIIT) – Pyramid (10-8-6-4-2 Reps)		Start with 10 reps of each, decrease by 2 each round until 2 reps.			
Inchworm	Core, Shoulders, Hamstrings	Walk hands forward to plank, hold, walk back to standing.			
Push-Up w/ Extension	Chest, Triceps, Core	Do push-up, extend one arm forward, alternate sides.			
Tuck Jumps	Legs, Core, Cardio	Jump explosively, tuck knees to chest mid-air, land softly.			
Workout No 264 (CrossFit) – 12-Minute AMRAP		Complete as many rounds as possible in 12 minutes.			
10 Step-Ups	Legs, Glutes, Core	Step onto raised surface, alternate legs, keep controlled movement.			
12 Spiderman Push-Ups	Chest, Core, Shoulders	Lower into push-up while bringing knee to elbow, alternate sides.			
15 Donkey Kicks	Glutes, Core, Balance	On hands and knees, kick leg back and up, squeeze glutes.			
Workout No 265 (HIIT) – 5-Minute Burnout Finisher		Perform 5 exercises continuously for 1 minute each. No rest.			
High Knees	Cardio, Core, Legs	Drive knees high, move fast, pump arms aggressively.			
Squats	Legs, Glutes, Core	Lower hips below knees, keep chest up, push through heels.			
Plank	Core, Shoulders, Endurance	Hold plank position, engage core, maintain straight line.			
Mountain Climbers	Core, Cardio, Shoulders	Run in place from plank, drive knees toward chest.			
Workout No 266 (CrossFit) – 12-Minute AMRAP (As Many Rounds As Possible)		Complete as many rounds as possible in 12 minutes. Move fast while maintaining good form.			
10 Burpees	Full Body, Core, Cardio	Jump, drop into a push-up, jump back up. Move fast and land softly.			
15 Squats	Legs, Glutes, Core	Lower hips below knees, push through heels to rise, keep chest up.			
20 Mountain Climbers	Core, Cardio, Shoulders	In plank, drive knees toward chest, move quickly but controlled.			
Workout No 267 (HIIT) – 30 30 Intervals (4 Rounds)		30 seconds of work, 30 seconds rest per exercise. 4 total rounds.			
Jumping Jacks	Cardio, Shoulders, Core	Jump feet apart while clapping hands overhead, return to start. Move fast.			
High Knees	Cardio, Core, Legs	Run in place, drive knees high, pump arms aggressively.			
Side-to-Side Push-Ups	Chest, Triceps, Core	Do a push-up, shift to one side, push up again. Switch sides.			
Bicycle Crunches	Core, Abs, Obliques	Lie back, twist torso, bring elbow to opposite knee, extend leg.			

Workout	Main Muscle Groups	Instructions	Day 1	Day 2	Day 3
Workout No 268 (CrossFit) – 4 Rounds for Time		Complete 4 rounds as fast as possible. Minimal rest.			
12 Box Jumps	Legs, Glutes, Cardio	Jump onto a box, land softly, step down. Keep core tight.			
10 Pike Push-Ups	Shoulders, Triceps, Core	From downward dog position, lower head to ground, push up.			
15 Walking Lunges	Legs, Glutes, Core	Step into deep lunge, push through heel to stand, alternate legs.			
20 Flutter Kicks	Core, Lower Abs, Hip Flexors	Lie flat, keep legs straight, alternate kicking up and down.			
Workout No 269 (HIIT) – 20-Minute Tabata (20s Work, 10s Rest, 8 Rounds Per Exercise)		Alternate between 2 exercises, 20 seconds work, 10 seconds rest. 8 rounds.			
Side Plank (Left)	Core, Obliques, Shoulders	Hold plank on one side, engage core, breathe steadily. Stay straight.			
Side Plank (Right)	Core, Obliques, Shoulders	Switch sides, keep hips lifted, core tight. Breathe evenly.			
Skater Squats	Legs, Glutes, Core	Balance on one leg, squat, touch opposite hand to foot, switch sides.			
Jumping Jacks	Cardio, Shoulders, Core	Jump feet apart, clap hands overhead, return to start. Maintain rhythm.			
Workout No 270 (CrossFit) – 15-Minute Ladder (Increasing Reps Each Round)		Start with 2 reps per exercise, increase by 2 each round until 15 minutes are up.			
Squats	Legs, Glutes, Core	Lower hips below knees, drive through heels, keep chest up.			
Triceps Push-Ups	Triceps, Chest, Core	Hands under shoulders, elbows tight, lower chest to ground, push up.			
Mountain Climbers	Core, Cardio, Shoulders	Drive knees toward chest, keep core tight, move fast.			
Workout No 271 (HIIT) – 10-Minute Burnout (No Rest, Max Effort)		Move continuously for 10 minutes, switch exercises every 45 seconds.			
Burpees	Full Body, Cardio, Core	Jump explosively, drop into push-up, jump back up, repeat.			
Push-Backs	Shoulders, Arms, Core	From push-up position, push hips back toward heels, return to plank.			
Russian Twists	Core, Obliques, Abs	Sit with feet lifted, twist torso side to side, touch ground beside hips.			
Workout No 272 (CrossFit) – 21-15-9 Rep Scheme		Complete 21 reps of each, then 15, then 9, as fast as possible.			
Burpees	Full Body, Cardio, Core	Drop into push-up, jump explosively, land softly, repeat.			
Reverse Crunch	Core, Lower Abs, Hip Flexors	Lift hips off floor, knees toward chest, control descent.			
Crab Toe Touch	Core, Shoulders, Coordination	In crab position, touch opposite hand to foot, switch sides.			

Workout	Main Muscle Groups	Instructions	Day 1	Day 2	Day 3
Workout No 273 (HIIT) – Pyramid (10-8-6-4-2 Reps)		Start with 10 reps of each, decrease by 2 each round until 2 reps.			
Inchworm	Core, Shoulders, Hamstrings	Walk hands forward to plank, hold, walk back to standing.			
Push-Up w/ Extension	Chest, Triceps, Core	Do push-up, extend one arm forward, alternate sides.			
Tuck Jumps	Legs, Core, Cardio	Jump explosively, tuck knees to chest mid-air, land softly.			
Workout No 274 (CrossFit) – 12-Minute AMRAP		Complete as many rounds as possible in 12 minutes.			
10 Step-Ups	Legs, Glutes, Core	Step onto raised surface, alternate legs, keep controlled movement.			
12 Spiderman Push-Ups	Chest, Core, Shoulders	Lower into push-up while bringing knee to elbow, alternate sides.			
15 Donkey Kicks	Glutes, Core, Balance	On hands and knees, kick leg back and up, squeeze glutes.			
Workout No 275 (HIIT) – 5-Minute Burnout Finisher		Perform 5 exercises continuously for 1 minute each. No rest.			
High Knees	Cardio, Core, Legs	Drive knees high, move fast, pump arms aggressively.			
Squats	Legs, Glutes, Core	Lower hips below knees, keep chest up, push through heels.			
Plank	Core, Shoulders, Endurance	Hold plank position, engage core, maintain straight line.			
Mountain Climbers	Core, Cardio, Shoulders	Run in place from plank, drive knees toward chest.			
Workout No 276 (CrossFit) – 12-Minute AMRAP (As Many Rounds As Possible)		Complete as many rounds as possible in 12 minutes. Move fast while maintaining good form.			
10 Burpees	Full Body, Core, Cardio	Jump, drop into a push-up, jump back up. Move fast and land softly.			
15 Squats	Legs, Glutes, Core	Lower hips below knees, push through heels to rise, keep chest up.			
20 Mountain Climbers	Core, Cardio, Shoulders	In plank, drive knees toward chest, move quickly but controlled.			
Workout No 277 (HIIT) – 30 30 Intervals (4 Rounds)		30 seconds of work, 30 seconds rest per exercise. 4 total rounds.			
Jumping Jacks	Cardio, Shoulders, Core	Jump feet apart while clapping hands overhead, return to start. Move fast.			
High Knees	Cardio, Core, Legs	Run in place, drive knees high, pump arms aggressively.			
Side-to-Side Push-Ups	Chest, Triceps, Core	Do a push-up, shift to one side, push up again. Switch sides.			
Bicycle Crunches	Core, Abs, Obliques	Lie back, twist torso, bring elbow to opposite knee, extend leg.			

Workout	Main Muscle Groups	Instructions	Day 1	Day 2	Day 3
Workout No 278 (CrossFit) – 4 Rounds for Time	Complete 4 rounds as fast as possible. Minimal rest.				
12 Box Jumps	Legs, Glutes, Cardio	Jump onto a box, land softly, step down. Keep core tight.			
10 Pike Push-Ups	Shoulders, Triceps, Core	From downward dog position, lower head to ground, push up.			
15 Walking Lunges	Legs, Glutes, Core	Step into deep lunge, push through heel to stand, alternate legs.			
20 Flutter Kicks	Core, Lower Abs, Hip Flexors	Lie flat, keep legs straight, alternate kicking up and down.			
Workout No 279 (HIIT) – 20-Minute Tabata (20s Work, 10s Rest, 8 Rounds Per Exercise)	Alternate between 2 exercises, 20 seconds work, 10 seconds rest. 8 rounds.				
Side Plank (Left)	Core, Obliques, Shoulders	Hold plank on one side, engage core, breathe steadily. Stay straight.			
Side Plank (Right)	Core, Obliques, Shoulders	Switch sides, keep hips lifted, core tight. Breathe evenly.			
Skater Squats	Legs, Glutes, Core	Balance on one leg, squat, touch opposite hand to foot, switch sides.			
Jumping Jacks	Cardio, Shoulders, Core	Jump feet apart, clap hands overhead, return to start. Maintain rhythm.			
Workout No 280 (CrossFit) – 15-Minute Ladder (Increasing Reps Each Round)	Start with 2 reps per exercise, increase by 2 each round until 15 minutes are up.				
Squats	Legs, Glutes, Core	Lower hips below knees, drive through heels, keep chest up.			
Triceps Push-Ups	Triceps, Chest, Core	Hands under shoulders, elbows tight, lower chest to ground, push up.			
Mountain Climbers	Core, Cardio, Shoulders	Drive knees toward chest, keep core tight, move fast.			
Workout No 281 (HIIT) – 10-Minute Burnout (No Rest, Max Effort)	Move continuously for 10 minutes, switch exercises every 45 seconds.				
Burpees	Full Body, Cardio, Core	Jump explosively, drop into push-up, jump back up, repeat.			
Push-Backs	Shoulders, Arms, Core	From push-up position, push hips back toward heels, return to plank.			
Russian Twists	Core, Obliques, Abs	Sit with feet lifted, twist torso side to side, touch ground beside hips.			
Workout No 282 (CrossFit) – 21-15-9 Rep Scheme	Complete 21 reps of each, then 15, then 9, as fast as possible.				
Burpees	Full Body, Cardio, Core	Drop into push-up, jump explosively, land softly, repeat.			
Reverse Crunch	Core, Lower Abs, Hip Flexors	Lift hips off floor, knees toward chest, control descent.			
Crab Toe Touch	Core, Shoulders, Coordination	In crab position, touch opposite hand to foot, switch sides.			

Workout	Main Muscle Groups	Instructions	Day 1	Day 2	Day 3
Workout No 283 (HIIT) – Pyramid (10-8-6-4-2 Reps)		Start with 10 reps of each, decrease by 2 each round until 2 reps.			
Inchworm	Core, Shoulders, Hamstrings	Walk hands forward to plank, hold, walk back to standing.			
Push-Up w/ Extension	Chest, Triceps, Core	Do push-up, extend one arm forward, alternate sides.			
Tuck Jumps	Legs, Core, Cardio	Jump explosively, tuck knees to chest mid-air, land softly.			
Workout No 284 (CrossFit) – 12-Minute AMRAP		Complete as many rounds as possible in 12 minutes.			
10 Step-Ups	Legs, Glutes, Core	Step onto raised surface, alternate legs, keep controlled movement.			
12 Spiderman Push-Ups	Chest, Core, Shoulders	Lower into push-up while bringing knee to elbow, alternate sides.			
15 Donkey Kicks	Glutes, Core, Balance	On hands and knees, kick leg back and up, squeeze glutes.			
Workout No 285 (HIIT) – 5-Minute Burnout Finisher		Perform 5 exercises continuously for 1 minute each. No rest.			
High Knees	Cardio, Core, Legs	Drive knees high, move fast, pump arms aggressively.			
Squats	Legs, Glutes, Core	Lower hips below knees, keep chest up, push through heels.			
Plank	Core, Shoulders, Endurance	Hold plank position, engage core, maintain straight line.			
Mountain Climbers	Core, Cardio, Shoulders	Run in place from plank, drive knees toward chest.			
Workout No 286 (CrossFit) – 12-Minute AMRAP (As Many Rounds As Possible)		Complete as many rounds as possible in 12 minutes. Move fast while maintaining good form.			
10 Burpees	Full Body, Core, Cardio	Jump, drop into a push-up, jump back up. Move fast and land softly.			
15 Squats	Legs, Glutes, Core	Lower hips below knees, push through heels to rise, keep chest up.			
20 Mountain Climbers	Core, Cardio, Shoulders	In plank, drive knees toward chest, move quickly but controlled.			
Workout No 287 (HIIT) – 30 30 Intervals (4 Rounds)		30 seconds of work, 30 seconds rest per exercise. 4 total rounds.			
Jumping Jacks	Cardio, Shoulders, Core	Jump feet apart while clapping hands overhead, return to start. Move fast.			
High Knees	Cardio, Core, Legs	Run in place, drive knees high, pump arms aggressively.			
Side-to-Side Push-Ups	Chest, Triceps, Core	Do a push-up, shift to one side, push up again. Switch sides.			
Bicycle Crunches	Core, Abs, Obliques	Lie back, twist torso, bring elbow to opposite knee, extend leg.			

Workout	Main Muscle Groups	Instructions	Day 1	Day 2	Day 3
Workout No 288 (CrossFit) – 4 Rounds for Time	Complete 4 rounds as fast as possible. Minimal rest.				
12 Box Jumps	Legs, Glutes, Cardio	Jump onto a box, land softly, step down. Keep core tight.			
10 Pike Push-Ups	Shoulders, Triceps, Core	From downward dog position, lower head to ground, push up.			
15 Walking Lunges	Legs, Glutes, Core	Step into deep lunge, push through heel to stand, alternate legs.			
20 Flutter Kicks	Core, Lower Abs, Hip Flexors	Lie flat, keep legs straight, alternate kicking up and down.			
Workout No 289 (HIIT) – 20-Minute Tabata (20s Work, 10s Rest, 8 Rounds Per Exercise)	Alternate between 2 exercises, 20 seconds work, 10 seconds rest. 8 rounds.				
Side Plank (Left)	Core, Obliques, Shoulders	Hold plank on one side, engage core, breathe steadily. Stay straight.			
Side Plank (Right)	Core, Obliques, Shoulders	Switch sides, keep hips lifted, core tight. Breathe evenly.			
Skater Squats	Legs, Glutes, Core	Balance on one leg, squat, touch opposite hand to foot, switch sides.			
Jumping Jacks	Cardio, Shoulders, Core	Jump feet apart, clap hands overhead, return to start. Maintain rhythm.			
Workout No 290 (CrossFit) – 15-Minute Ladder (Increasing Reps Each Round)	Start with 2 reps per exercise, increase by 2 each round until 15 minutes are up.				
Squats	Legs, Glutes, Core	Lower hips below knees, drive through heels, keep chest up.			
Triceps Push-Ups	Triceps, Chest, Core	Hands under shoulders, elbows tight, lower chest to ground, push up.			
Mountain Climbers	Core, Cardio, Shoulders	Drive knees toward chest, keep core tight, move fast.			
Workout No 291 (HIIT) – 10-Minute Burnout (No Rest, Max Effort)	Move continuously for 10 minutes, switch exercises every 45 seconds.				
Burpees	Full Body, Cardio, Core	Jump explosively, drop into push-up, jump back up, repeat.			
Push-Backs	Shoulders, Arms, Core	From push-up position, push hips back toward heels, return to plank.			
Russian Twists	Core, Obliques, Abs	Sit with feet lifted, twist torso side to side, touch ground beside hips.			
Workout No 292 (CrossFit) – 21-15-9 Rep Scheme	Complete 21 reps of each, then 15, then 9, as fast as possible.				
Burpees	Full Body, Cardio, Core	Drop into push-up, jump explosively, land softly, repeat.			
Reverse Crunch	Core, Lower Abs, Hip Flexors	Lift hips off floor, knees toward chest, control descent.			
Crab Toe Touch	Core, Shoulders, Coordination	In crab position, touch opposite hand to foot, switch sides.			

Workout	Main Muscle Groups	Instructions	Day 1	Day 2	Day 3
Workout No 293 (HIIT) – Pyramid (10-8-6-4-2 Reps)		Start with 10 reps of each, decrease by 2 each round until 2 reps.			
Inchworm	Core, Shoulders, Hamstrings	Walk hands forward to plank, hold, walk back to standing.			
Push-Up w/ Extension	Chest, Triceps, Core	Do push-up, extend one arm forward, alternate sides.			
Tuck Jumps	Legs, Core, Cardio	Jump explosively, tuck knees to chest mid-air, land softly.			
Workout No 294 (CrossFit) – 12-Minute AMRAP		Complete as many rounds as possible in 12 minutes.			
10 Step-Ups	Legs, Glutes, Core	Step onto raised surface, alternate legs, keep controlled movement.			
12 Spiderman Push-Ups	Chest, Core, Shoulders	Lower into push-up while bringing knee to elbow, alternate sides.			
15 Donkey Kicks	Glutes, Core, Balance	On hands and knees, kick leg back and up, squeeze glutes.			
Workout No 295 (HIIT) – 5-Minute Burnout Finisher		Perform 5 exercises continuously for 1 minute each. No rest.			
High Knees	Cardio, Core, Legs	Drive knees high, move fast, pump arms aggressively.			
Squats	Legs, Glutes, Core	Lower hips below knees, keep chest up, push through heels.			
Plank	Core, Shoulders, Endurance	Hold plank position, engage core, maintain straight line.			
Mountain Climbers	Core, Cardio, Shoulders	Run in place from plank, drive knees toward chest.			

Body-Weight Exercises

Alternate Arm/Leg Plank

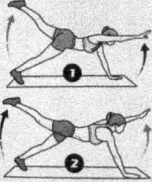

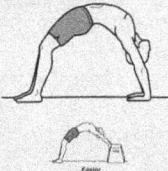

Plank, extend opposite arm and leg, hold.

1. Start in a plank position with hands directly under shoulders.
2. Simultaneously lift and extend your right arm and left leg.
3. Hold this position for a few seconds.
4. Return to the plank position.
5. Repeat with the left arm and right leg.

Army Crawl

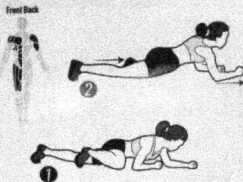

Crawl flat on stomach, using elbows and knees.

1. Lie flat on your stomach with elbows bent and hands directly in front of you.
2. Push with your toes and pull with your elbows to crawl forward.
3. Keep your body low and hips down.
4. Continue crawling for the desired distance or time.

Back Bridge

Plank, extend opposite arm and leg, hold.

1. Lie on your back with knees bent and feet flat on the floor.
2. Place your hands palms down by your sides.
3. Press through your feet and lift your hips up towards the ceiling.
4. Hold this position, squeezing your glutes and keeping your core tight.
5. Lower your hips back down to the starting position.

Bear Crawl

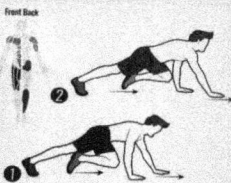

Crawl forward on all fours, hips down, move quickly.

1. Start on all fours with hands under shoulders and knees under hips.
2. Lift your knees slightly off the ground, keeping your back flat.
3. Move your right hand and left foot forward simultaneously.
4. Follow with your left hand and right foot, maintaining a low position.
5. Continue moving forward in this manner quickly.

Bicycle Crunches

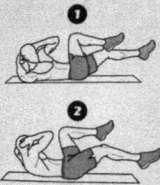

Lie down, alternate elbows to opposite knees cycling legs.

1. Lie on your back with hands behind your head and knees bent.
2. Lift your shoulders off the ground and bring your right elbow towards your left knee while extending the right leg.
3. Switch sides, bringing your left elbow towards your right knee while extending the left leg.
4. Continue alternating sides in a pedaling motion.

Bird Dog

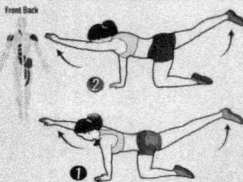

Extend opposite arm and leg, kneeling position.

1. Start on all fours with hands under shoulders and knees under hips.
2. Extend your right arm forward and your left leg backward simultaneously.
3. Hold for a few seconds, keeping your core engaged.
4. Return to the starting position.
5. Repeat with the left arm and right leg.

Bodyweight Row

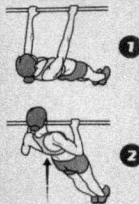

Pull body up towards a bar or table, lying underneath.

1. Position yourself under a bar or table, gripping it with both hands.
2. Keep your body straight and pull your chest up towards the bar.
3. Hold for a moment at the top of the movement.
4. Lower yourself back down to the starting position.
5. Repeat for the desired number of repetitions.

Burpee

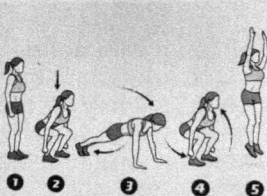

Jump, squat down, kick back into a push-up, return up.

1. Start standing with feet shoulder-width apart.
2. Drop into a squat position and place your hands on the ground.
3. Kick your feet back into a push-up position and lower your body to the ground.
4. Push back up to the push-up position and jump your feet back to your hands.
5. Explosively jump into the air, reaching your arms overhead.
6. Land softly and repeat.

Calf Raise

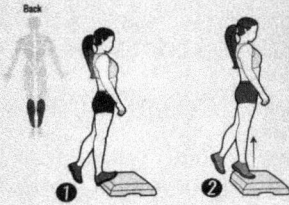

Raise heels off ground, balance on toes, lower slowly.

1. Stand with feet hip-width apart on a flat surface or step.
2. Lift your heels off the ground, balancing on the balls of your feet.
3. Hold the position for a second.
4. Slowly lower your heels back to the ground.
5. Repeat for the desired number of repetitions.

Calf Raises

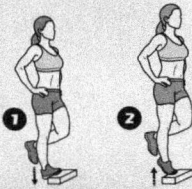

Lift heels off ground, balance on toes, lower slowly.

1. Stand with feet hip-width apart on a flat surface or step.
2. Lift your heels off the ground, balancing on the balls of your feet.
3. Hold the position for a second.
4. Slowly lower your heels back to the ground.
5. Repeat for the desired number of repetitions.

Cat/Camel

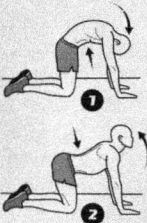

On hands and knees, arch back up and down.

1. Start on all fours with hands under shoulders and knees under hips.
2. Arch your back up towards the ceiling (Cat position).
3. Hold for a few seconds.
4. Lower your back down and lift your head and tailbone up (Camel position).
5. Alternate between the two positions, moving slowly and smoothly.

Crab Toe Touch

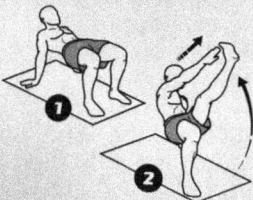

Crawl forward on all fours, hips down, move quickly.

1. Sit on the ground with knees bent, feet flat, and hands behind you.
2. Lift your hips off the ground into a crab position.
3. Reach your right hand to touch your left foot while lifting it.
4. Return to the starting position.
5. Repeat with the left hand and right foot, alternating sides.

Crab Walk

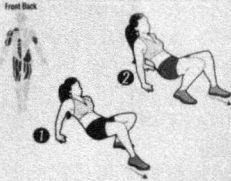

Walk backward on hands and feet, hips elevated.

1. Sit on the ground with knees bent, feet flat, and hands behind you.
2. Lift your hips off the ground into a crab position.
3. Walk backward using your hands and feet, keeping hips elevated.
4. Continue for the desired distance or time.

Crocodile Crawl

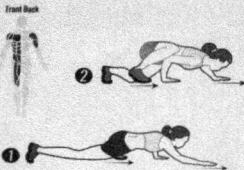

Crawl forward lying almost flat, use elbows and toes.

1. Start in a plank position with elbows bent and body low to the ground.
2. Move forward by simultaneously pulling with one arm and pushing with the opposite leg.
3. Keep your body as low and flat as possible.
4. Continue crawling forward for the desired distance or time.

Cross-Body Crunch

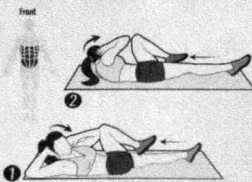

Touch opposite knee to elbow, lying down.

1. Lie on your back with knees bent and hands behind your head.
2. Lift your shoulders off the ground and bring your right elbow towards your left knee while extending the right leg.
3. Return to the starting position.
4. Repeat with the left elbow towards the right knee, alternating sides.

Crunch

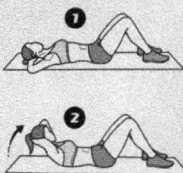

Lift shoulders off ground, contract abdominals.

1. Lie on your back with knees bent and feet flat on the ground.
2. Place your hands behind your head without pulling on your neck.
3. Lift your shoulders off the ground by contracting your abdominal muscles.
4. Hold for a second at the top.
5. Slowly lower back down to the starting position.

Dolphin Kick

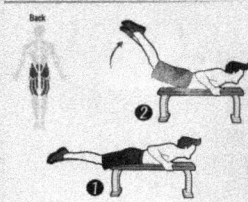

Lie face down, kick legs like a dolphin's tail.

1. Lie face down on a bench with your hips at the edge.
2. Hold onto the bench for support.
3. Lift your legs off the ground, keeping them straight.
4. Kick your legs up and down like a dolphin's tail.
5. Continue for the desired number of repetitions or time.

Donkey Kicks

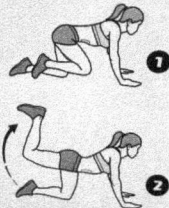

On hands and knees, kick one leg back and up.

1. Start on all fours with hands under shoulders and knees under hips.
2. Keep your right knee bent and lift your right leg up towards the ceiling.
3. Squeeze your glutes at the top.
4. Lower your leg back down without touching the ground.
5. Repeat on the other leg.

Fire Hydrant

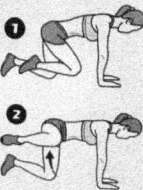

On hands and knees, lift leg to side, keep knee bent.

1. Start on all fours with hands under shoulders and knees under hips.
2. Keep your right knee bent and lift it out to the side.
3. Hold for a moment at the top.
4. Lower your knee back down without touching the ground.
5. Repeat on the other leg.

Flutter Kicks

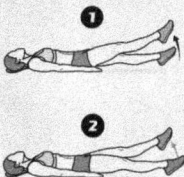

Lie on back, alternately kick legs in small, rapid motion.

1. Lie on your back with hands under your hips for support.
2. Lift both legs off the ground slightly.
3. Alternately kick your legs up and down in a small, rapid motion.
4. Keep your core engaged and back flat on the ground.
5. Continue for the desired time.

Glute Bridge

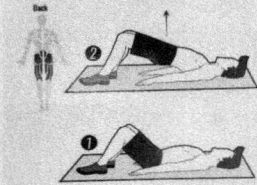

Lift hips while lying on back, feet flat on ground.

1. Lie on your back with knees bent and feet flat on the ground.
2. Place your arms by your sides with palms down.
3. Lift your hips towards the ceiling by squeezing your glutes.
4. Hold for a moment at the top.
5. Lower your hips back to the starting position.

Good Morning

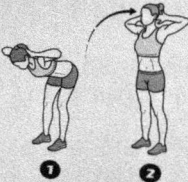

Hinge at hips with hands behind head, focus on hamstrings.

1. Stand with feet shoulder-width apart and hands behind your head.
2. Keep your back straight and hinge at the hips, bending forward.
3. Lower your torso until it's parallel to the ground.
4. Focus on feeling the stretch in your hamstrings.
5. Return to the starting position by engaging your glutes and hamstrings.

Hanging Knee Raise

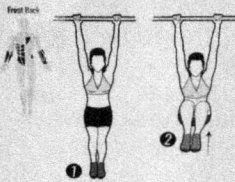

Hang from bar, raise knees towards chest.

1. Hang from a bar with arms extended and feet off the ground.
2. Keep your legs straight and together.
3. Lift your knees towards your chest by engaging your core.
4. Hold for a moment at the top.
5. Lower your legs back to the starting position.

High Knees

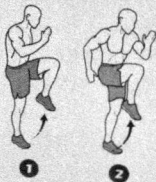

Run in place lifting knees high, maintain pace.

1. Stand with feet hip-width apart.
2. Run in place, lifting your knees as high as possible.
3. Pump your arms in coordination with your legs.
4. Maintain a quick pace and keep your core engaged.
5. Continue for the desired time.

Hip Raise

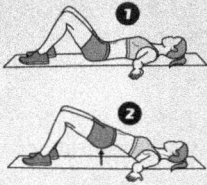

Lift hips while lying on back, feet flat on ground.

1. Lie on your back with knees bent and feet flat on the ground.
2. Place your arms by your sides with palms down.
3. Lift your hips towards the ceiling by squeezing your glutes.
4. Hold for a moment at the top.
5. Lower your hips back to the starting position.
6. Repeat for the desired number of repetitions.

Inchworm

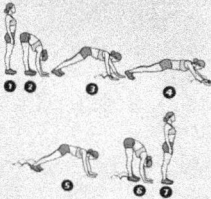

Walk hands forward from standing, hold plank, walk back.

1. Stand with feet hip-width apart.
2. Bend at the waist and place your hands on the ground.
3. Walk your hands forward until you are in a plank position.
4. Hold the plank for a few seconds.
5. Walk your hands back towards your feet and stand up.
6. Repeat for the desired number of repetitions.

Jumping Jacks

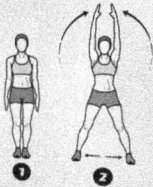

Jump to spread legs and clap hands overhead.

1. Stand with feet together and arms at your sides.
2. Jump to spread your legs while raising your arms overhead to clap.
3. Jump back to the starting position with feet together and arms at your sides.
4. Maintain a quick pace and keep your movements controlled.
5. Repeat for the desired number of repetitions or time.

Leg Pull-In

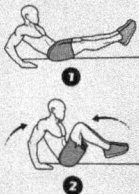

Sit, pull knees into chest, extend legs out.

1. Sit on the ground with legs extended and hands behind you for support.
2. Lean back slightly and lift your legs off the ground.
3. Pull your knees into your chest.
4. Extend your legs back out without touching the ground.
5. Repeat for the desired number of repetitions.

Lunge

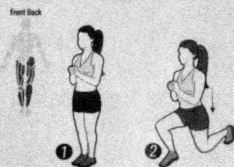

Step forward, lower hips to drop knee to ground.

1. Stand with feet hip-width apart.
2. Step forward with your right leg and lower your hips to drop your right knee towards the ground.
3. Ensure your right knee is directly above your ankle.
4. Push through your right heel to return to the starting position.
5. Repeat with the left leg, alternating sides.

Lying Leg Lift

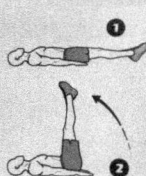

Raise legs vertically, lying flat on back.

1. Lie flat on your back with legs extended and arms by your sides.
2. Keep your legs straight and lift them towards the ceiling until they form a 90-degree angle with your torso.
3. Hold for a moment at the top.
4. Lower your legs back down without touching the ground.
5. Repeat for the desired number of repetitions.

Mountain Climber

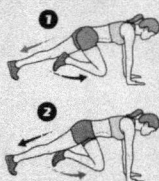

Run in place in plank position, drive knees to chest.

1. Start in a plank position with hands under shoulders and body in a straight line.
2. Bring your right knee towards your chest.
3. Quickly switch legs, bringing your left knee towards your chest while extending your right leg back.
4. Continue alternating legs in a running motion.
5. Maintain a quick pace and keep your core engaged.

Pike Push Up

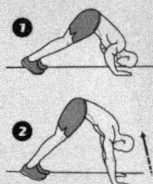

Push-up with hips high, resembles downward dog pose.

1. Start in a downward dog position with hips high and hands shoulder-width apart.
2. Lower your head towards the ground by bending your elbows.
3. Push through your hands to return to the starting position.
4. Keep your body in an inverted V shape throughout the movement.
5. Repeat for the desired number of repetitions.

Plank Rotation

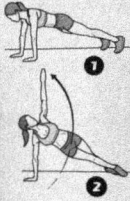

Rotate body in plank, extend arm upward, switch sides.

1. Stand with feet hip-width apart.
2. Step forward with your right leg and lower your hips to drop your right knee towards the ground.
3. Ensure your right knee is directly above your ankle.
4. Push through your right heel to return to the starting position.
5. Repeat with the left leg, alternating sides.

Pull Up

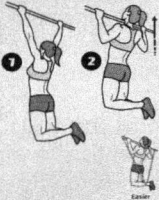

Pull body up on bar, chin above hands.

1. Hang from a pull-up bar with hands shoulder-width apart and palms facing away.
2. Engage your core and pull your body up until your chin is above the bar.
3. Hold for a moment at the top.
4. Lower yourself back down to the starting position with control.
5. Repeat for the desired number of repetitions.

Push Up

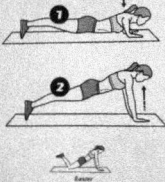

Lower body to ground, push up with arms.

1. Start in a plank position with hands slightly wider than shoulder-width apart.
2. Lower your body towards the ground by bending your elbows.
3. Keep your body in a straight line from head to heels.
4. Push through your hands to return to the starting position.
5. Repeat for the desired number of repetitions.

Push-Back

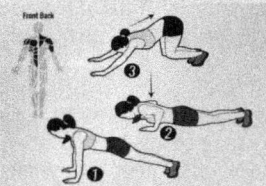

Push body back from push-up position to heels.

1. Start in a plank position with hands under shoulders.
2. Push your hips back towards your heels while keeping your arms extended.
3. Lower your chest towards the ground.
4. Return to the starting plank position.
5. Repeat for the desired number of repetitions.

Push-Up w/ Extension

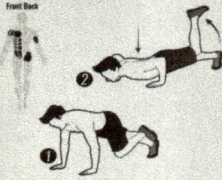

Perform push-up, extend one
arm forward, alternate.

1. Start in a plank position with hands under shoulders.
2. Perform a push-up by lowering your body to the ground.
3. As you push back up, extend your right arm forward.
4. Return your hand to the ground.
5. Repeat with the left arm, alternating sides.

Reverse Crunch

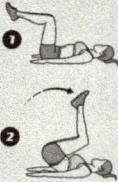

Lift hips off floor, knees
towards chest.

1. Lie on your back with knees bent and feet flat on the ground.
2. Place your hands by your sides or under your hips for support.
3. Lift your hips off the ground and bring your knees towards your chest.
4. Hold for a moment at the top.
5. Lower your hips back to the starting position.
6. Repeat for the desired number of repetitions.

Reverse Plank

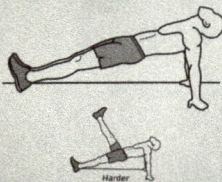

Sit, lift body with arms, legs
straight, face up.

1. Sit on the ground with legs extended and hands behind you, fingers pointing forward.
2. Lift your hips off the ground by pressing through your hands and heels.
3. Keep your body in a straight line from head to heels.
4. Hold for the desired time.
5. Lower your hips back to the ground.

Russian Twist

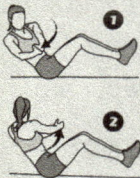

Twist torso holding weight,
seated on ground.

1. Sit on the ground with knees bent and feet flat.
2. Lean back slightly and lift your feet off the ground, balancing on your sit bones.
3. Hold a weight with both hands and twist your torso to the right, bringing the weight beside your hip.
4. Twist to the left, bringing the weight to the other side.
5. Continue alternating sides for the desired number of repetitions.

Scissor Kick

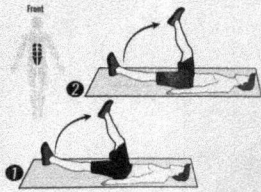

Alternately lift legs in lying position, engages core.

1. Lie flat on your back with hands under your hips for support.
2. Lift your legs slightly off the ground.
3. Alternately lift one leg higher while lowering the other leg, keeping both legs straight.
4. Continue the scissor motion, engaging your core throughout.
5. Repeat for the desired number of repetitions or time.

Side Crunches

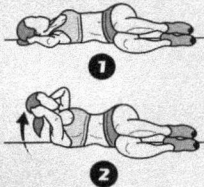

Lie on side, perform crunches towards elevated leg.

1. Lie on your side with legs bent and hands behind your head.
2. Lift your upper body towards your hips, crunching towards the elevated leg.
3. Squeeze your obliques at the top of the movement.
4. Lower back down to the starting position.
5. Repeat for the desired number of repetitions, then switch sides.

Side Lunge

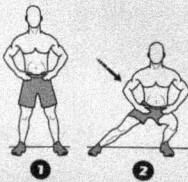

Step to side into lunge, keep other leg straight.

1. Stand with feet hip-width apart.
2. Step to the side with your right leg, lowering your hips into a lunge.
3. Keep your left leg straight and your chest up.
4. Push through your right foot to return to the starting position.
5. Repeat on the other side, alternating legs.

Side Plank

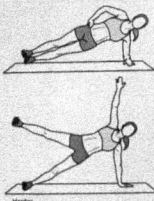

Support body on one arm, side facing ground.

1. Lie on your side with your elbow directly under your shoulder.
2. Lift your hips off the ground, forming a straight line from head to feet.
3. Hold this position, keeping your core engaged.
4. For added difficulty, extend your top arm towards the ceiling.
5. Repeat on the other side.

Side-to-Side Pull-Up

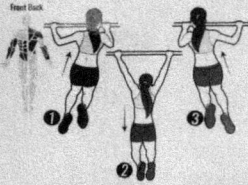

Pull up and move sideways along bar, alternate sides.

1. Hang from a pull-up bar with hands shoulder-width apart.
2. Pull your body up towards the bar, moving to the right side.
3. Lower yourself back down and pull up again, moving to the left side.
4. Continue alternating sides.
5. Repeat for the desired number of repetitions.

Side-to-Side Push-Up

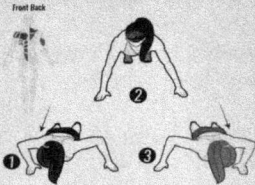

Shift side-to-side during push-ups, engages core.

1. Start in a plank position with hands slightly wider than shoulder-width apart.
2. Lower your body towards the ground, shifting your weight to the right.
3. Push back up and shift your weight to the left.
4. Continue alternating sides with each push-up.
5. Repeat for the desired number of repetitions.

Single Leg Dead Lift

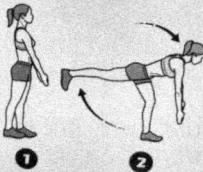

Balance on one leg, hinge forward, extend free leg back.

1. Stand on your right leg with a slight bend in the knee.
2. Hinge at the hips, extending your left leg back and lowering your torso towards the ground.
3. Keep your back straight and core engaged.
4. Return to the starting position by squeezing your glutes.
5. Repeat on the other leg, alternating sides.

Single Leg Split Squat

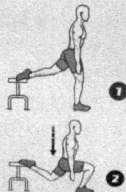

Perform split squat on one leg, elevated rear foot.

1. Stand a few feet in front of a bench or elevated surface.
2. Place your right foot behind you on the bench.
3. Lower your hips into a squat, keeping your left knee over your ankle.
4. Push through your left heel to return to the starting position.
5. Repeat on the other leg, alternating sides.

Single Leg Squat

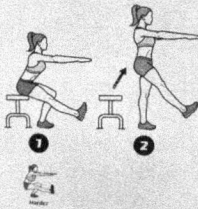

Stand on one leg, squat, maintain balance.

1. Stand on your right leg, extending your left leg in front.
2. Lower your hips into a squat, keeping your left leg elevated.
3. Maintain balance and keep your chest up.
4. Push through your right heel to return to the starting position.
5. Repeat on the other leg, alternating sides.

Skater Squat

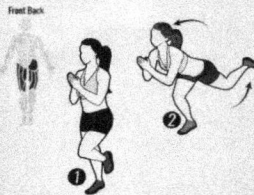

Balance on one leg, squat, touch opposite hand to foot.

1. Balance on your right leg, bending your left knee.
2. Lower into a squat while reaching your left hand towards your right foot.
3. Keep your back straight and chest up.
4. Push through your right heel to return to the starting position.
5. Repeat on the other leg, alternating sides.

Spiderman

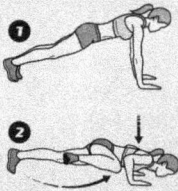

Bring knee to elbow during push-up, switch sides.

1. Start in a push-up position with hands under shoulders.
2. Lower your body towards the ground while bringing your right knee to your right elbow.
3. Push back up to the starting position.
4. Repeat with the left knee to the left elbow, alternating sides.
5. Continue for the desired number of repetitions.

Squat

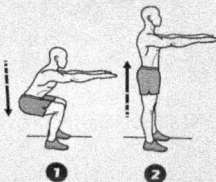

Stand, bend knees to lower body, keep back straight.

1. Stand with feet shoulder-width apart and arms extended in front.
2. Bend your knees and lower your hips into a squat.
3. Keep your back straight and chest up.
4. Push through your heels to return to the starting position.
5. Repeat for the desired number of repetitions.

Star Plank

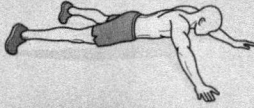

Extend arms and legs out from body in plank position.

1. Start in a plank position with hands under shoulders and feet together.
2. Extend your right arm and left leg out to the sides.
3. Hold for a moment, keeping your core engaged.
4. Return to the starting position and repeat with the left arm and right leg.
5. Alternate sides for the desired number of repetitions.

Step Up

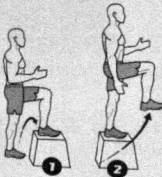

Step onto a raised platform, alternate legs.

1. Stand in front of a raised platform or bench.
2. Step up with your right foot, bringing your left knee towards your chest.
3. Step back down with your left foot, then your right foot.
4. Repeat with the left foot leading, alternating sides.
5. Continue for the desired number of repetitions.

Stretching

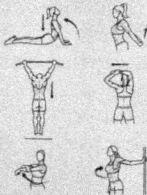

Perform various stretches to improve flexibility and cool down.

1. Perform a variety of stretches, targeting all major muscle groups.
2. Hold each stretch for 15-30 seconds.
3. Focus on slow, controlled movements to increase flexibility.
4. Include stretches for the hamstrings, quadriceps, calves, chest, back, and shoulders.
5. Ensure a thorough cool-down to aid in recovery.

Sumo Squat

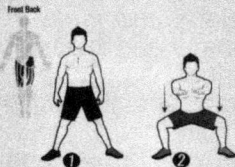

Wide stance squat, toes pointed out, lower body.

1. Stand with feet wider than shoulder-width apart and toes pointed out.
2. Lower your hips into a squat, keeping your back straight and chest up.
3. Ensure your knees track over your toes.
4. Push through your heels to return to the starting position.
5. Repeat for the desired number of repetitions.

Superman

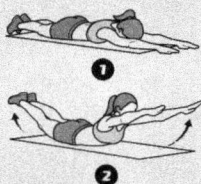

Extend arms and legs while face down, hold position.

1. Lie face down on the ground with arms extended forward and legs straight.
2. Lift your arms, chest, and legs off the ground simultaneously.
3. Hold the top position for a few seconds.
4. Lower back down to the starting position.
5. Repeat for the desired number of repetitions.

Swimmer

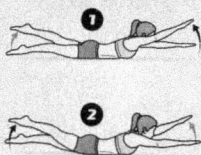

Lie face down, alternate lifting arms and legs.

1. Lie face down on the ground with arms extended forward and legs straight.
2. Lift your right arm and left leg off the ground simultaneously.
3. Lower them back down and lift your left arm and right leg.
4. Continue alternating sides in a swimming motion.
5. Repeat for the desired number of repetitions or time.

Tricep Dip

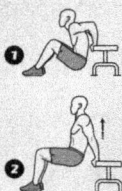

Dip body between bars, focus on triceps.

1. Sit on the edge of a bench or chair with hands gripping the edge.
2. Slide your hips off the edge, supporting your weight with your arms.
3. Lower your body by bending your elbows to a 90-degree angle.
4. Push through your palms to return to the starting position.
5. Repeat for the desired number of repetitions.

Tricep Push Up

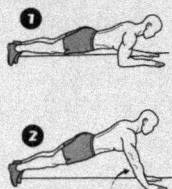

Push-up with hands under shoulders, elbows tight.

1. Start in a plank position with hands under shoulders and elbows close to your body.
2. Lower your body towards the ground, keeping elbows tight to your sides.
3. Push through your palms to return to the starting position.
4. Keep your body in a straight line throughout the movement.
5. Repeat for the desired number of repetitions.

Tuck Jumps

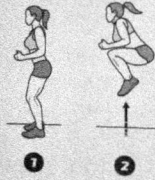

Jump high, tuck knees to chest mid-air.

1. Stand with feet hip-width apart and knees slightly bent.
2. Jump explosively, bringing your knees towards your chest.
3. Land softly on the balls of your feet with knees slightly bent.
4. Immediately jump again, maintaining quick, controlled movements.
5. Repeat for the desired number of repetitions or time.

V Up

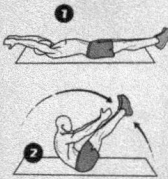

Lie back, lift legs and torso simultaneously, form 'V'.

1. Lie on your back with arms extended overhead and legs straight.
2. Simultaneously lift your legs and torso off the ground, reaching your hands towards your feet.
3. Form a "V" shape with your body at the top of the movement.
4. Lower back down to the starting position with control.
5. Repeat for the desired number of repetitions.

Walking Lunge

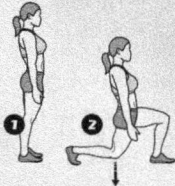

Step forward into a lunge, move forward alternating legs.

1. Stand with feet hip-width apart and hands on your hips.
2. Step forward with your right leg, lowering into a lunge.
3. Push through your right heel to stand and bring your left leg forward into the next lunge.
4. Continue alternating legs, moving forward with each step.
5. Repeat for the desired number of repetitions or distance.

Walking Toe Touches

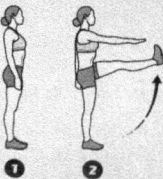

Walk, reach down to touch toes with opposite hand.

1. Stand with feet hip-width apart.
2. Step forward with your right leg, lifting it straight in front of you.
3. Reach your left hand to touch your right toes.
4. Lower your leg and step forward with your left leg, reaching your right hand to your left toes.
5. Continue alternating sides as you walk forward.

Wall Sit

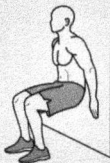

Sit against wall, legs at 90 degrees, hold position.

1. Stand with your back against a wall.
2. Slide down the wall until your thighs are parallel to the ground.
3. Keep your feet shoulder-width apart and knees at a 90-degree angle.
4. Hold this position for the desired amount of time.
5. Maintain tension in your thighs and keep your back flat against the wall.

Wall Squat

Front Back

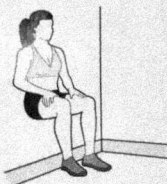

Lie face down, alternate lifting arms and legs.

1. Stand with your back against a wall, feet shoulder-width apart.
2. Slide down into a squat position, keeping your back against the wall.
3. Ensure your thighs are parallel to the ground and knees are above your ankles.
4. Hold this position for the desired time.
5. Maintain proper form by keeping your back straight and core engaged.

Wide/Narrow Push Up

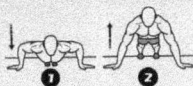

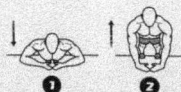

Perform push-ups with varying hand widths.

1. Start in a plank position with hands wider than shoulder-width apart.
2. Lower your body to the ground by bending your elbows.
3. Push through your palms to return to the starting position.
4. Move your hands closer together, directly under your shoulders.
5. Perform another push-up in this narrow position.
6. Alternate between wide and narrow push-ups for the desired repetitions.

Windshield Wiper

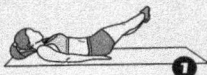

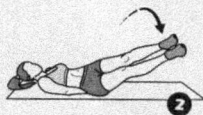

Swing legs side-to-side lying down, mimic wiper.

1. Lie on your back with arms extended out to the sides for support.
2. Lift your legs off the ground and bring them to a 90-degree angle.
3. Slowly lower your legs to the right side, keeping them together.
4. Bring your legs back to the center.
5. Lower your legs to the left side.
6. Continue alternating sides, mimicking a windshield wiper motion.

www.ingramcontent.com/pod-product-compliance
Lightning Source LLC
Chambersburg PA
CBHW032102020426
42335CB00011B/458